On Hope and Healing

**For Those Who Have Fallen
Through the Medical Cracks**

Et Alia Series in Writing and Wellness, Volume 1.

For book orders and inquiries, contact
    Gordon Medical Associates
    3471 Regional Parkway
    Santa Rosa, California 95403

    Email neil@gordonmedical.com

Published in the United States of America by
    Et Alia Press
    5001 Woodlawn Drive
    Little Rock, Arkansas 72205

ISBN 978-0-9828184-0-4
Library of Congress Control Number   2010931219

Text edited by Casey D. White
Cover and text layout by Valerie Kidd Turner and Jesse Nickles
Anatomical drawings by Carla Stine

Cover: Morning Sun in Orr Hot Springs, Northern California. Photograph by Neil Nathan.

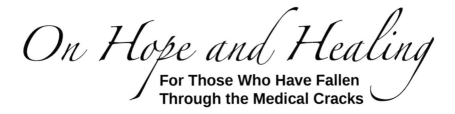

On Hope and Healing
For Those Who Have Fallen
Through the Medical Cracks

by Neil Nathan, M.D.

Pritzker School of Medicine, University of Chicago

Foreword by Jacob Teitelbaum, M.D.

Edited by Casey D. White
Iowa State University

Printed in conjunction with
Gordon Medical Associates
Santa Rosa, California

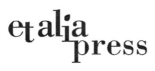

Little Rock, Arkansas

2010

I promised, many, many years ago, that if I ever wrote a book, that I would dedicate it to my beloved wife, Cheryl. I love the word "dedication." It not only fulfills my promise, but it also describes our incredible relationship. She is my muse, my inspiration, support and nurturance, and without her I strongly suspect that this book would not have come into being. Thank you, from the bottom, middle, and top of my heart.

Contents

FOREWORD

Although the rest of the planet is moving into the twenty-first century, most of our health care system is fixed firmly in a well out-of-date past. This book describes how having an open mind and an intellectual curiosity, combined with a compassionate heart, can turn an M.D. physician into a cutting-edge holistic physician. This journey can also teach you the tools that can help you reclaim your health—even when your standard physician mistakenly believes that there is "nothing that can be done."

And Then Came Dr. Nathan . . .

A funny thing happens when a bright, well-educated physician sees treatments work that medically are not supposed to (e.g. hypnosis, chiropractic, herbals). As Winston Churchill once said, "We often stumble over the truth. Fortunately, we usually manage to get up, brush ourselves off, and walk away quickly before any real harm is done." But Dr. Nathan didn't walk away quickly enough . . .

In a world where most doctors only hear about the newest and most expensive (and also most toxic) treatments, Neil Nathan has discovered that medicine has lost its way. Having found that numerous natural, safe, and inexpensive therapies work far better than prescriptions, he has dedicated his life to applying these discoveries for his patients' well being. Though he tends to be easygoing, helping those patients that found their way to him was not enough. His caring and compassion has driven him to help as many as he can. So he decided to write this book.

Hope

Frustrated with how medicine has become a cold assembly line? Hopeless that your doctor will ever truly understand you, or the impact your illness is having? Given up on finding a doctor that can actually help you?

Dr. Nathan's book shows you that there is hope, as well as what is possible in medicine and in a caring medical practice.

He starts where a doctor should—at the beginning. What are the simple and most critical nutrient and hormonal deficiencies? Magnesium deficiency, for example, can be presumed to be present in most Americans, and causes unnecessary suffering and debility, as well as way too many premature deaths. The average American gets less than 300 mg of magnesium a day vs. over 600 mg in a standard Chinese diet, because of the magnesium losses in food processing. At a nickel a day, encouraging magnesium supplementation is not glamorous—but it could easily save your life. He recognizes hormonal deficiencies are also running rampant, and are usually missed by our incredibly inaccurate lab testing. He then tells you what you need to know to take care of these problems. Having a doctor who recognizes and starts with the basics is a real gift!

From these basics, Dr. Nathan will take the reader into new worlds of ideas and inspirations that most physicians will never open their minds to—simply because they are cheap and simple, and, therefore, there is no money to encourage their being taught at the big pharmaceutical advertising orgies we call "scientific medical conferences."

What happens then is no less than magical. Illnesses and problems that your physician said were incurable (and sometimes not even diagnosable) become clearly understood, with the path laid out for your reclaiming your health!

Along the way, you will find that Dr. Nathan gives many personal stories about how the treatments he discusses have helped individual patients. Knowing Dr. Nathan well, I know he does this for a very simple reason. He takes his patients', and now his readers', wellbeing very personally.

I think you will enjoy reading this book. When you are done, you will enjoy reclaiming your health—and a life you love!

Love and Blessings,

Jacob Teitelbaum, M.D.
Kona, Hawaii
14 February 2009

An Open Letter to Readers

*I*f you have been suffering with an undiagnosed illness or are struggling with a named illness and are not improving (or are actually worsening, despite the best efforts of your healthcare providers), I have written this book for you.

If you are a physician or healthcare provider and have become aware that you are not helping as many of your patients as you might have hoped, I have written this book for you, too.

The early beginnings of *On Hope and Healing* grew out of a three-day course that I developed and taught to fellow physicians, which I called "What Every Physician Should Know about Treating Complex Illness." It was my hope that I could simplify, and make practical, the emergent discipline of "functional medicine," so that doctors who were newly exposed to this information could take it back with them to their offices and start using this material to help patients.

After a time, I realized that this course material could be the foundation for a book that might also help my more motivated patients to better understand their illnesses—and, in turn, to make better medical decisions. This body of information grew steadily, evolving into the book that you now hold in your hand.

There are as many ways to read this book as there are physicians' and patients' needs. A patient might choose to read from cover to cover or pick-and-choose from the Table of Contents or proceed to the Appendix, which lists patients' stories regarding specific illnesses. (If you suffer, say, from fibromyalgia or chronic fatigue, you might take these patients' stories as a starting point; you might then look up the illness and treatments in the Index and proceed accordingly.)

Before elaborating further, I wish to invite my Et Alia series editor, Dr. James S. Baumlin, to share his thoughts on this book and its aims. Addressing patients primarily, his words appear in italics below.

Whereas open letters of this sort are rarely written in tandem, whole books do arise out of conversations and collaborations. Dr. Nathan's textual editor, Casey D. White, has done his part, so I suppose it's my turn to contribute a little something to the cause.

I have overseen the publication of On Hope and Healing *out of an unwavering conviction that books can save lives, and that a physician's best prescription includes information—reading— as well as medication. For, you see, I was Dr. Nathan's patient before I was his press editor. I was among those many unfortunate who had "fallen through the medical cracks," showing a series of seemingly inscrutable neurological symptoms that Dr. Nathan eventually diagnosed as mold toxicity—a medical condition that, in my case, developed full-blown into multiple chemical sensitivities (MCS). The latter diagnosis seemed a prison sentence to me, since MCS is a debilitating condition for which conventional (allopathic) medicine offers no viable treatment. As I sat slouched in his office, reeling from the building's disinfectants (which worked upon my weakened nervous system like so many poisons), Dr. Nathan scanned his bookshelves. Eventually his eyes fell upon a book whose homeopathic subject was "allergy elimination," a notion that Western medicine finds implausible, though Eastern "alternative" medicine takes it for granted.*

"Another patient of mine found this book helpful," he said, standing and pulling it from the shelf. "Read it and see what you think."

Read it I did, and put it to practice; as a consequence, my MCS symptoms—while not cured—have subsided, becoming more an inconvenience than a disability. I have, in effect, gotten my life back. And I owe this to a book recommended to me by an open-minded holistic practitioner. Most other physicians in my purview would not have heard, much less have read, of the protocols described therein: had they heard of it, many would have been incredulous, some mistrustful, a few downright hostile. To illustrate, let me tell a brief story.

When Dr. Nathan moved his practice from Springfield, Missouri (my hometown) to Santa Rosa, California, I felt very much alone but not yet desperate. I had researched my various conditions, after all, and could write up my own narrative "case history," including a summary-record of medications, protocols and treatments. Armed with this written narrative, I made an appointment with a well-respected local practitioner—I'll call him Dr. M—in hopes that he might become my family physician. His terse response has been seared into my memory.

"I don't know what that is," he said, referring to something in my narrative. "I wouldn't prescribe that," he added, referring to some medication or other. "That's not part of my paradigm," he concluded, referring vaguely to one of the illnesses, perhaps, or to one of the treatments. "Is there anything else I can help you with?" were his final, dismissive words. I left his office less in anger than in shock.

What did my little episode with Dr. M teach me? That the typical allopath is not well equipped to diagnose, much less to treat, many of the complex/chronic illnesses assaulting this current generation. The typical allopath will not have heard of some treatments listed in this book; worse, he or she might not believe in the disease itself. I wish I had had the presence of mind to ask Dr. M which of my treatments were "not part" of his precious "paradigm."

I do know that many physicians question the very existence of mold toxicity; perhaps that was why Dr. M neglected to prescribe a medication as safe and simple as cholestyramine (which aids in removing micotoxins from the body). Also— despite recent research to the contrary—much of the medical profession holds fast to the notion that MCS is not physiological but psychological in origin: that is, it's all "in the patient's head."

Admittedly, mold and MCS are my own bugbears. I admire the courage of colleagues who raise autistic children, and I have watched them search, often frantically, for answers: "How, why did this happen?" "What do we do now?" Working from academic studies (often underwritten by pharmaceutical, chemical, and insurance companies), the scientific community still refuses to acknowledge that incidents of autism have risen exponentially over recent decades. "The data do not support claims that autism is on the rise. In the past, incidents went unreported, whereas now they are often misdiagnosed and misreported." So goes the typical lecture that the typical nursing student hears in a typical college classroom in America. Given such "official" attitudes, the parent of an autistic child will feel very much alone—as will the person suffering from mold toxicity or MCS or fibromyalgia or chronic fatigue. If you as a patient (or a patient's family member) find yourself feeling similarly "on your own," the information in this book should give you hope. But don't be surprised if you have to teach your physician some of what you'll have learned; and don't be too surprised if your physician misunderstands, disapproves, or chooses not to listen. ("That's not part of my paradigm . . . .")

While I no longer care to see Dr. M, I am fortunate to have met Dr. S. Though diffident upon hearing my story—"I don't know if I can help you," was his initial response—Dr. S. rose to the occasion. "I don't know if I can help you," he said, adding, "but I'll try." What more can one ask? Dr. S. has never "rubber stamped" a protocol or a medication that I've brought to his attention; he exercises a healthy skepticism and does his own homework, and I trust his judgment. Together, we are becoming a team, and I am grateful for that fact.

I should add that I am fortunate and grateful for having been Dr. Nathan's one-time patient. Let me say, too, that the above remarks are my own entirely, unsolicited and not necessarily a reflection of Dr. Nathan's views. I would never, ever recommend that ideas presented in this book be pursued against the advice (or without the knowledge and consent) of an individual's personal physician. My aim in writing as a patient to other patients—indeed, in writing of complex/chronic illness to others facing similar circumstances—is to affirm the necessary collaboration between a patient and his or her healthcare practitioners; this is a collaboration best built upon trust, shared responsibility, active research, and honest communication.

At this point, I yield the floor back to Dr. Nathan, who shall address physicians' concerns and further ways of reading this book.

By virtue of the fact that you hold this book in your hand, you are distinguishing yourself from the run-of-the-mill practitioner whose "paradigm" does not embrace holistic treatment and alternative therapies. Those of you who are just starting your own practice or want to make improvements to your current care-giving model might begin at the beginning and proceed systematically from there. Since this book presents my philosophy in action, it starts with the most basic topics: How does one create a nonthreatening, comforting office environment? How does one treat one's patients—that is, not their illnesses per se, but their persons, learning to listen, to respect, to inform, and to empathize as well as to diagnose and heal?

As with my course materials, I have organized this book in the sequence that I deemed most beneficial for those who are new to holisitic practices. But many of you will already be "on board" and looking for alternative treatments to your patients' chronic/complex illnesses. I trust that the book's "apparatus" (the Table of Contents, Appendix, and Index) will lead you to the "chapter and verse" that will prove of most service. But let me add a further piece of advice. Do share the information in this book—better yet, share this book, along with others in your library—with those patients who take an active interest in their illness and in the means of healing.

As Dr. Baumlin suggests above, I keep a lending library in my medical office and have never hesitated to prescribe reading as well as medication. Our profession would be performing a great, humane service if it recommitted to educating and not simply to treating patients, as if the means of treatment were so many mysteries imparted secretively to a priestly caste. Let us all agree not to fall into this aggrandizing delusion, which places the patient beneath us rather than beside us as partners in their healing.

For the wise practitioner knows that healing comes from within the patient, and that we caregivers can best serve as midwives to that healing. Over my career, I have learned that the single greatest asset that a patient (and a physician) can possess is hope. A patient without hope will rarely heal; a patient with hope has a very good chance. This book, thus, is on hope and healing, in that right order. By gathering together the latest diagnostic and treatment techniques and organizing them into a coherent whole, this book aims to serve those many thousands who, sadly, have "fallen through the medical cracks." Its practical treatments give a real basis for hope: there is good reason to hope, even in the midst of chronic/complex illness, and this book gives the proof.

Regardless of how you approach this material, it is my deepest wish that this book be valuable to you. Enjoy, and be well!

Neil Nathan, M.D.
Santa Rosa, California
14 July 2010

James S. Baumlin, Ph.D.
Springfield, Missouri
14 July 2010

Introduction

A Book of Hope

Welcome to my world! It is filled with hope, especially for those of you who have "fallen through the medical cracks." Let me explain what I mean by this.

Many of you have seen multiple health practitioners: doctors, chiropractors, naturopaths, massage therapists, physical therapists, and psychologists. Most of you have tried really hard and spent a great deal of time and money and effort to feel better or to get an explanation for your symptoms. Perhaps you've already surfed the internet, attempting to sift through a tremendous amount of information, only to become utterly confused by the contradictory opinions from site to site. If you're lucky in your personal research, you might be a little better or perhaps just treading water, or maybe you're slowly but steadily getting worse.

My practice is composed almost entirely of patients just like you. How that happened is a somewhat long story, and I'll tell that story in the first few chapters of this book. For now, however, I'd simply like to clarify the message that holds together not only this book, but also my entire practice, the entire reason that I do what I do. That message is hope. To understand the concepts that can create this hope, we first need to understand the kinds of medical diagnoses and treatments that you have already been offered—you know, the ones that aren't working.

Those concepts and treatments are based on an old and somewhat simplistic idea that each disease has one cause and therefore one specific treatment. This is a delightful idea, and when it works it makes medicine enjoyable to practice and yields wonderful results. Doctors' responses to many medical conditions reflect this model: we diagnose strep throat with a throat culture and treat it with penicillin; we diagnose iron deficiency anemia with a blood test and treat it with iron; we diagnose blockage of the coronary arteries with an arteriogram and treat it with a coronary balloon or stint or with bypass surgery, depending on the specifics. This model of conventional medicine has been in place for the last 150 years, and it is still taught in medical schools and practiced by nearly all physicians.

The problem for many of you, unfortunately, is that most chronic illnesses are not caused by a single event or imbalance, but by a complex interrelationship between multiple body systems. To treat them, consequently, requires a new model, one which embraces this complexity and strives to understand and appreciate it. Understanding fatigue, for example, requires that we comprehend how the adrenal gland, thyroid gland, sex hormones, magnesium metabolism, and the digestive and immune systems all intertwine. Identifying and fixing just one piece of the problem (which would mean adhering to the old model) often leads to temporary improvement, but the body just can't sustain that improvement. The remaining unidentified imbalances and deficiencies override the temporary improvement, and people go back to being fatigued. To heal this fatigue requires some patience and a detailed understanding of the intricate relationship among all the possible causes. It also requires a knowledge of how these factors work together to create this fatigue in this patient at this exact moment in time. That is what this book is about.

In our current managed health care system, when only a quick visit to the doctor's office is allotted, your primary care physician cannot begin to address the magnificent complexity of your body. Those of you who are insured in this fashion are permitted brief, unsatisfying visits and are quickly told after a short while that all of your symptoms are probably psychological in origin. You emerge with the impression that because your physician has a limited amount of time to work with you, she doesn't quite know what to do about any of the symptoms you are having. You would be right.

After months or years of regular medical visits with no answers, no improvement, and no real treatment offered, who wouldn't become frightened and depressed? You've been wrestling with feeling truly awful for a long time, and then you are told that medical science has absolutely no explanation for your illness. This adds another dimension to your illness, but it's not the cause, and until we identify the cause(s) and treat them, you cannot get well.

From my medical perspective, the essence of healing is about diagnosis—finding out why you are not well. Without a clear diagnosis, we have no viable starting point from which we can evaluate your illness and treat it. In a nutshell, a clear diagnosis is crucial to beginning any treatment program; without it, we are just guessing, and how likely are we to be of help if we are just shooting in the dark?

Here's where I part ways from some of my colleagues in medicine. I am convinced that a more precise diagnosis is available for my patients using this new body of knowledge, which I will convey to you in this book. Unfortunately, it appears that most physicians are not aware of this information. The reason I am filled with hope is because I have treated thousands of patients in this manner and have seen wonderful successes. My purpose in writing this book is to help you understand a large body of information that has been acquired over the past twenty years by a group of pioneering physicians, each of whom has recognized the limitations of the current medical model and has found useful, new fields of knowledge to expand upon that model. I am honored to be a part of that group of physicians and to have the opportunity to convey to you what we've been learning. These fields provide us with much of the information we need to accurately put together the complexity of your imbalances and address their treatment in an organized manner.

In the first few chapters of this book, I will describe my own personal journey of discovery, how I learned to put all of this together. I will identify six major imbalances common to most of my long-suffering patients, and I call them the "Big Six." These are imbalances of the adrenal gland, thyroid, sex hormones, magnesium, food allergy, and overgrowth of yeast and toxic bacteria in the intestinal tract. Each of these imbalances has its own chapter and will be dealt with in detail.

In the next group of chapters, I will discuss some of the less common imbalances, which I call the "Little Six." These include heavy metal toxicity (especially mercury); residual infections such as the Epstein-Barr virus (mononucleosis), Lyme disease, and mycoplasma infections; mold toxicity; amino acid deficiencies; hypoglycemia; and the newly identified central biochemical deficiencies of methylation chemistry. Although these imbalances are less common than those in the "Big Six", they are nevertheless significant contributors to illness and must be addressed. Please understand that there are many more imbalances than the twelve emphasized here. It is not my intention to be encyclopedic in this discussion, but rather to focus on what I believe to be the most practical common areas for evaluation and treatment. While I know that some of this information is somewhat technical, I will make every effort to explain these imbalances as clearly as possible so you can begin to understand the bigger picture of how all of these biochemical concepts interface with each other.

Over a few more chapters, we will take a detailed look at pain so that we can learn how to be more specific and comprehensive in both diagnosis and treatment. This will include a discussion of the fields of prolotherapy and osteopathic manipulation as examples of under-appreciated treatments.

Finally, I will try to synthesize all of this information and discuss the emotional and spiritual components of illness. Why are we seeing such an explosion of these unusual illnesses at this time in history? Hopefully this book will bring us closer to some answers to that important question.

I am honored to have Jacob Teitelbaum, M.D., a pioneer in the treatment of fibromyalgia and chronic fatigue, comment on this new model in his Foreword to this book. We believe it will help many of you to recover your health.

Welcome to a new vision of what is possible in the realms of healing.

❖ ❖ ❖

Acknowledgments

First, I would like to express my deepest thanks to Dr. James S. Baumlin, Professor of English at Missouri State University. Jim took his fledgling writer/physician, who had only completed a few chapters of a book, and encouraged, coaxed, prodded, and thoroughly supported that effort through its completion.

Next, I wish to express my gratitude to Casey D. White, who spent long days and nights converting my efforts into a completed manuscript and never seemed to tire of keeping me on track. Thanks, I needed that!

Special thanks go to Valerie Turner for her artistic vision and patience with all of my last-minute changes that went into the creation of this book; for her efforts I am deeply appreciative.

I also thank Jesse Nickles, who put the finishing touches on the book's layout and cover art.

Without the dedication and commitment and caring of my fabulous Springfield, Missouri staff, Neva Dix and Kevin Joyce, this work would not be possible. The pursuit of healing requires a team effort, and I could not have had a better team covering my back at all times.

Now that my family and I have moved to northern California, I am part of a new team at Gordon Medical Associates, and I am grateful to

Eric Gordon, M.D., my friend and colleague, as well as his associates, Win Bertrand, M.D., Wayne Anderson M.D., P.A., and Justin Cauntay, D.O., who have continued my education and reviewed this manuscript for us.

Thanks, too, to my brother, Gene Nathan, M.D., and to Gene Shippen, M.D., Jacob Teitelbaum, M.D., and Ritchie Shoemaker, M.D., for their support, assistance, brilliance, and inspiration, but most of all for their friendship.

And last, but never least, I wish to thank my patients, one and all, for their patience, hard work, and willingness to teach me everything they know. While medical science has many opinions about how to approach illness, my patients carry the truth of their responses to our treatment efforts with them, and that is where learning really happens.

My heart overflows with gratitude to all of you.

Further Disclaimers

As excited as I hope you will be to try the treatments we describe, please understand that all of them, under some circumstances, present some risk or danger to you or your family. *Please do not embark on any treatment without the assistance of someone who is medically trained, knowledgeable, and experienced in the details of the testing and treatment programs we describe.*

This book is not intended to be used as a treatment manual, but rather as a starting point for understanding your illness and a catalyst for initiating the progress of your medical journey.

Throughout this book, with a few exceptions which are clearly noted, I have changed the names of the patients who have consented to have their case histories presented here. I am doing so to protect their privacy, but know that I have taken care to present their medical information as accurately as possible.

As medical information evolves, so does the work in progress that represents our life stories. By the time this book has gone into print, some of the details of medical information may have changed, along with some of the stories that reflect my patients' histories. What you read in this volume is the best, most current truth that I have access to at this time, subject to change at a moment's notice. I will do my utmost to stay at the cutting edge of those truths.

Photo Credits

Cover: Morning Sun in Orr Hot Springs, Northern California. Photograph by Neil Nathan.

Page xxvi: Clay Pots, Kuleto Winery, Northern California. Photograph by Cheryl Nathan.

Page 12: Cherry Blossoms, Mendocino Botanical Gardens. Photograph by Cheryl Nathan.

Page 56: Tiger Swallowtail on Lilac Bush. Photograph by Cheryl Nathan.

Page 100: Ice Plants and Ocean, Mendocino Botanical Gardens. Photograph by Cheryl Nathan.

Page 114: Redwoods in Morning Sunshine. Photograph by Neil Nathan.

Page 126: Camelia in the Foreground of Redwoods. Photograph by Neil Nathan.

Page 152: White Mountains of New Hampshire. Photograph by Neil Nathan.

Page 178: Early Morning on Navarro Ridge. Photograph by Cheryl Nathan.

Page 188: Pacific Ocean near Dragonfly Cottage, Trinidad, California (with special thanks to Jeanine Martin). Photograph by Neil Nathan.

Page 218: "Falling Through the Not-So Medical Cracks": Pacific Ocean near Dragonfly Cottage (close-up of ocean scene on page 188). Photograph by Neil Nathan.

Page 240: Rhododendron, Mendocino Botanical Gardens. Photograph by Cheryl Nathan.

Page 264: Dogwood Blossoms. Photograph by Cheryl Nathan.

Page 286: Neil Nathan with his Puppy Kai on Isla Mujeres, Mexico. Photograph by Cheryl Nathan.

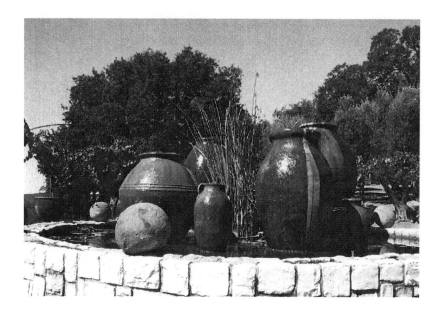

Chapter 1

Falling through the Medical Cracks

I am a physician. But when people ask me what I do for a living, I find it very difficult to answer, not because I don't know, but because what I actually do for patients isn't a part of conventional medical practice and doesn't yet have a name. Over time, I started to describe my work as treating patients who have "fallen through the medical cracks," a phrase that seems to resonate with my patients. I also describe my practice as "complex medical problem solving," and I actually think of myself as a sort of medical detective who discovers the causes for the illnesses of those patients who seek me out, most often because they've not found what they needed elsewhere in terms of healing. The vast majority of these patients have seen multiple physicians and other healthcare practitioners before they make it to my doorstep.

This field of medicine has evolved slowly over my thirty-eight years of medical practice. Initially, as a family physician, I provided the full range of medical services: I delivered babies and took care of them afterward, completed some minor surgeries, took my share of protracted shifts in the emergency room, and for many years was up all hours of the day and night providing the best medical care I could. Despite excellent training at both the University of Chicago Pritzker School of Medicine and San Francisco General Hospital, I encountered many patients whom

I could not adequately help with my available knowledge and skills. I slowly began to realize that my education had not entirely prepared me for all of the difficult problems I had to deal with in patients, day-in and day-out. So I began to look for answers elsewhere.

One of my first partners was a superb chiropractor, Stan Weisenberg, who, in 1974, at a time when chiropractors and medical doctors typically didn't associate, took the time to teach me the rudiments of manipulative medicine. *Manipulative medicine* is simply a fancy phrase used to describe the use of hands-on treatments to alleviate a wide variety of aches and pains. Under Stan's careful guidance, I conducted my first neck-cracking procedure, absolutely terrified that I might do something wrong. For those of you who have not experienced this procedure, it involves the patient lying on her back while the treating healthcare provider cradles the neck with both hands. The patient's neck is rapidly turned to the side in a carefully orchestrated but sudden motion, a maneuver often associated with a distinct cracking sound and/or sensation, which is intended to free up a vertebra that is jammed or stuck.

Over time, I began to appreciate the precision and the palpatory skills necessary to conduct these procedures, and also to both diagnose and treat difficult musculoskeletal problems. I developed a deep admiration for those engaged in this work. As time moved on, I studied with osteopathic physicians, chiropractors, massage therapists, and physical therapists, all of whom used somewhat different approaches that were helpful for certain health care problems. I soon began to discover that there was not one specific branch of medicine that had all of the answers; rather, each field of study provided its own set of clues and information that helped to solve the more complicated cases. Sometimes I refer to these skills and new areas of information as my "bag of tools," and I have found that with each addition to that bag, I am able to help more and more patients.

Around the time I began working with manipulative medicine, I ran into a situation that would forever change the way I looked at illness. During my studies at the University of Chicago School of Medicine, I took an elective course in medical hypnosis, merely because it sounded interesting. While the material fascinated me, I just didn't have the opportunity to see how hypnosis could be used successfully in clinical practice. So I filed the information somewhere in the storage rooms in the back of my mind. After completing my internship and a wonderful tour with the Indian Health Service in South Dakota, Oklahoma, and Alaska, I went to Mendocino, a small town in northern California, to begin my medical practice. I often worked in the emergency room of our local hospital, and within a few months, a woman presented to us with a severe asthma attack. I admitted her and tried every known conventional treatment to try to improve her breathing. A consultant agreed that we were doing everything possible to help her, but she continued to pant and gasp uncontrollably, and her labored respirations were exhausting her. Desperate to find something helpful, I poured through the books in our hospital library and found a single sentence in a medical textbook casually suggesting that hypnosis could sometimes be useful for treating severe bronchospasms.

At that time, my knowledge and experience of hypnosis were rudimentary and crude, limited simply to that elective class I took in medical school. I could hardly envision this frantic and breathless woman following my finger with her eyes as I slowly attempted to lead her into a state of relaxation. Nevertheless, I explained to her what I wanted to do, and with no other visible options, we resolved to try. In the most soothing voice I could conjure (considering that I was almost as frightened by her condition as she), I asked her to follow my finger as I slowly moved it back and forth across her eyes and gently led her through a basic relaxation exercise. To my astonishment, within fifteen minutes her breathing had calmed considerably, her wheezing and panting subsided, and she was now breathing almost normally. I had not imagined that this result was possible. She did extremely well following our single session and was able to leave the hospital the next day.

I continued to work with this patient using hypnosis, and as we explored the causes for her asthma attack, she confessed that her breathing difficulties began when she learned that her son was going to marry a woman she did not approve of. As she began to process and adjust to this stressful situation, her health improved steadily. Keep in mind that this was 1974, and nowhere in my medical training had it been suggested that intense stress could produce this sort of illness. The reality of this information was staring me right in the face: here was a potentially invaluable tool, hypnosis, a procedure that could open new doors to understanding and treating illness that I never dreamed existed. I realized immediately that I had to learn a great deal more about how to work with this tool, so I read everything I could get my hands on about hypnosis and discovered that it had a long tradition of proven value in the treatment of a wide variety of medical conditions: headaches, anxiety, depression, bed wetting, and low back pain, among others. I began to explore its use whenever I ran into a medical situation where my customary tools were ineffective.

Several months later, a woman named Paula came into my office with severe rheumatoid arthritis and peptic ulcer disease. These were somewhat related illnesses, since the medications used to treat her rheumatoid arthritis (anti-inflammatory medications and steroids) often cause stomach irritation, which can directly lead to ulcers. By this time, I had acquired a great deal more skill and confidence with hypnosis, which enabled patients to discover the relationship between specific stressors and their illnesses. In fact, Paula could vividly recall, under hypnosis, the exact moment when her illness had begun. Several years before, she had owned a chain of hair salons in Reno, Nevada. One day while she was working, an elegantly dressed woman came in with a doting family in tow. This client had severe rheumatoid arthritis with classically deformed joints in her hands, and although she had great difficulty moving, her family waited on her every need as she received her salon treatment. Paula recalled feeling deeply, wistfully jealous of this woman, and in her own successful but lonely life, wished that she, too, could be taken care of in this loving manner. Within a few weeks, Paula noted the onset of joint pain, and within a year she had developed full-blown rheumatoid arthritis. She became disabled and had to sell her chain of salons. She eventually moved to a small town north of Mendocino, purchasing a small motel that she ran with the help of others.

Paula had become increasingly disabled by the time she sought my help. Her excruciating ulcers were preventing her from taking the typical medications used to treat her arthritis, so with no other options known to me at that time, I offered the use of hypnosis to explore and treat her illness. She agreed. As we noted earlier, while she was under hypnosis, Paula learned fairly quickly how her illness had begun, and we explored the longing for care that had triggered these events. But how was I to treat it? As I explored her illness, it became obvious that she was holding on to a great deal of suppressed emotion, which pre-dated her arthritis. While she was hypnotized, I offered her the oppor-tunity to allow herself to both feel and express those emotions. Over several subsequent sessions, Paula wept and sobbed and raged, releas-ing all of her pent up emotions into the quiet solace of my office. To my amazement, she immediately began to improve. Not only did she improve, but her illness disappeared completely. All traces of rheuma-toid arthritis were gone, her blood tests came back to normal, and, most astonishingly, the joints of her hands completely healed. She was now able to stack cases of soda for the vending machines at her motel without difficulty, a task which would have previously been inconceivable.

I had frequently read in my medical textbooks that once the joints of the hands had deteriorated to this extent, healing was *impossible*. This should give you an idea of the magnitude of this change. There I was, looking at the impossible. There seemed to be a clear cause and effect here: the emotional events of Paula's life led directly to her development of an incapacitating physical disease. By understanding this process, I was able to, in a sense, reverse her disease. Nowhere in my medical education had anyone suggested that this was possible.

That singular event raised within me the obvious questions: How did this healing happen? What else is possible? Can this work for oth-ers with similar diseases? Can it work for others with different medical conditions? What other conditions are amenable to this approach? A whole new world had opened for me and I could not imagine leaving it unexplored.

Since rheumatoid arthritis is in the autoimmune disease family, I began to offer my patients with those diagnoses the option of exploring their illnesses with hypnosis. A few were a bit leery of the unconven-tionality of hypnosis as a treatment, but many took me up on it. Over the next several years, I treated more than a dozen patients using the process of hypnosis to explore the cause and treatment of their illnesses, and half of them were completely healed; their laboratory work returned to normal, and all manifestations of their disease vanished. While it is well known that autoimmune disease can occasionally go into spontaneous remission for no clear reason, my results were well beyond occasional and anything but spontaneous. In effect, this was well beyond anything that I had studied in conventional medicine. One of the most important things I learned was that it wasn't enough for patients to recall the traumatic or stressful origins of their illness. Until they actually *released* the stressful emotions held within their tissues, healing didn't seem to occur. But even when they did release these emotions, not everyone got well. Why not?

The practice of hypnosis initiated my understanding of the "mind-body connection" or its fancier but expressive name *psychoneuroimmunology*. There was a profound relationship between the stressors of my patients' lives—the burdens on their psyches—and the physical illnesses which manifested within them.

Shortly, another very different group of patients came to my attention. The first of these was sixteen-year-old Kevin, who was referred to me from a group-care home where he was residing. He had been afflicted with intractable grand mal seizures (in which the entire body shakes) for a number of years, and these seizures were poorly controlled by his medication. He'd seen multiple neurologists and had tried everything available, so again I was left with the only tool I could think of to help him: hypnosis.

Kevin was agreeable to exploring his seizures, so under hypnosis I asked him to relive the last few seizures, moment-by-moment. Every one of his episodes seemed to be triggered by intense emotion, either fear or rage. This was, again, a surprise. I had always been led to understand that seizures were caused by random electrical discharges in the brain, but these did not seem to be random. Since Kevin's seizures seemed directly related to how he dealt with intense emotions, this suggested the possibility of a specific treatment. I reasoned that if Kevin could control his fear or rage before it precipitated a seizure, maybe we could actually prevent them.

Under hypnosis, I taught Kevin how to recognize and take seriously the intensity of his emotions so that we could use a simple technique to control them. When previously working with asthma, I had learned a technique in which patients match the intensity of their bronchospasm to the tension level in their clenched fist. When they were able to match those tension levels precisely and have control over them, they would slowly, very slowly, open their fist. As the tension in their fist dissipated, the spasm in the bronchial muscles eased as well. This turned out to be a very effective tool in the treatment of asthma. I used the same concept with Kevin's seizures. I asked him to match his emotional intensity to the tension in his fist, and when he had control over his clenched fist, he could slowly let it open, simultaneously letting go of the emotional tension as well. This worked surprisingly well, and Kevin rapidly gained control over his seizures to the point that he was able to get off all medications and eliminate his seizures completely, all within the period of less than a year.

My success with Kevin prompted the referral of seven more youngsters with seizures. Again, when regressed under hypnosis to the moment of their last seizures, each reported intense fear or anger. These seizures were starting to look less like random events and more like predictable responses to overwhelming emotions. Over the course of the next year, half of these seizure patients were able to get off all medication, and the other half were better controlled on less medication.

Thinking I had just made a brand-new, wonderful discovery, I was primed to educate the medical world about this fabulous new treatment opportunity. Alas, I discovered that Sigmund Freud had described this same process in 1908! Although this was not the revolutionary breakthrough I had imagined it to be, it was still exciting and interesting to me. As intrigued as I was about these successful experiences, I was more surprised that my colleagues weren't just as thrilled. When I attempted to share with them what I had learned, most of them seemed to become uncomfortable hearing me talk about hypnosis and the importance of emotional release to its success. I'd expected from them the same kind of wonder or awe that I felt, but instead I found doubt, cynicism, and general disinterest. I had now come upon one of the most unexpected and difficult problems of all: How can I instill willingness in my fellow practitioners to listen to new information?

I did find a willing ear from my chiropractic mentor, Stan Weisenberg, who not only seemed to understand my experiences, but had himself been studying the effects of emotional release therapy on healing. He, in turn, introduced me to a wonderful Reichian therapist, Phil Curcurutto, who taught me even more about emotional release in healing, but this time from a different perspective. Dr. Curcurutto had studied directly with Dr. Wilhelm Reich, a physician who developed a technique using breathing, coupled with certain movements and massage, to facilitate the release of emotions. Utilizing these techniques in my practice deepened my awareness and knowledge of the connection between emotion and illness. Dr. Curcurutto had learned of another healing process, a technique called *osteopathic craniosacral manipulation,* which was not available for study to chiropractors (only to physicians, both osteopathic and allopathic, and dentists). He urged me to pursue that field of study.

This led to a trip to Colorado Springs in 1975 to study this new area. Osteopathic craniosacral manipulation is a branch of classical osteopathy, but at that time I had no idea what an osteopath was and I was simply going on my teacher's recommendation. So I wound up as the only M.D. in a room of osteopathic physicians, studying a new and obscure branch of healing. This technique, which we'll discuss in more detail later, requires an extremely light touch and an exquisite sense of palpation, neither of which I had at that time. Fortunately, the teaching faculty, perhaps the most incredible group of healers I had ever encountered, was very kind to me. They led me step by step to the perception of the "cranial rhythm" and its use. After three days of intense training, in which I had demonstrated no perceptual grasp of the rhythm, Dr. Edna Lay took pity on me and guided my awareness into recognition of the subtle cranial motions, for which I will always be grateful.

This experience profoundly changed my awareness of and ability to feel imbalances in the body and help heal them. Learning these techniques required a deeper study of anatomy than I had received in my traditional medical education, so my understanding of musculoskeletal problems improved dramatically, as well. Perhaps most important was the deep feeling of satisfaction that came from using my own hands to help relieve a patient's pain. It is always a source of wonder that once I've finished working on someone's neck or back or shoulders, the pinched look in his or her eyes is gone, there is a sense of peace or relaxation about the patient, and we have built a little more trust between us, which is a nice foundation for further healing. As my understanding of healing began to grow, this model of treatment began to expand in other directions. What I've described so far sounds like a nice integration of emotional, spiritual, and structural components of healing. And it is. But there was more to come.

At one of the first meetings of the American Holistic Medical

Association, I was fortunate to meet Dr. Robert Anderson from the state of Washington. During one of our discussions, Bob casually commented on how important it was to look for hidden food allergies in complicated patients. As he was then President of the American Holistic Medical Association, my respect for him was such that I immediately began to evaluate patients for unsuspected food allergies and found this to be far more common than I had been taught in medical school.

At about the same time, Drs. Orren Truss and William Crook started publishing material on intestinal yeast (*Candida*) infections as another major contributor to poor health. This idea opened up yet another field for my study and treatments. By the mid 1980s, hypoglycemia (low blood sugar) emerged as another missing piece of this puzzle. It was fascinating, too, watching how conventional medicine declined to embrace this information. Traditional medical teaching simply denied that looking for food allergy, intestinal yeast infections, and hypoglycemia were valid fields of study, despite the fact that when patients were examined and treated for these conditions, they clearly improved.

I began to see a curious process of polarization occurring among practitioners in my field: they had begun to take sides on how to look at these patients who presented to us with unexplained fatigue, fibromyalgia, headaches, depression, anxiety, and cognitive impairment. Conventional medicine continued to insist that these patients were psychologically impaired, and had no physical component to their illness, while some of us were seeing something else entirely. Traditional physicians had come to believe that stress, which was mostly psychological in nature, caused almost every symptom we couldn't explain in our patients, and for their anxiety or depression they needed either medication or counseling— or both. Those of us working in this new arena saw these so-called psychological problems disappear entirely when the correct diet, the correct supplements, and the correct biochemical corrections were prescribed. It was increasingly clear that the illnesses of these patients were not just in their heads, but in their body chemistry, as well. It was apparent that we had a lot more to learn about chemistry.

By the early 1990s, pioneering work by Dr. Norman Shealy and others had established that adrenal weakness (Chapter 3) and magnesium deficiency (Chapter 4) were major components to most chronic illnesses. Dr. Denis Wilson had begun to develop his concepts of thyroid deficiency with a unique approach (Chapter 5). Newer laboratory testing enabled us to accurately measure food allergies for the first time (Chapter 7). Additionally, we began to realize that chronic infections played a significant role in weakening the body. This idea had already been described by Dr. Jay Goldstein in the mid 1980s with his work on Epstein-Barr viral infections (EBV), but again, that work was quickly dismissed by conventional medicine. We began to document that other viruses, along with EBV, may contribute to this, especially Cytomegalovirus and HHV-6 (Chapter 12). The whole family of mycoplasma infections (including atypical or walking pneumonia) and Lyme disease (Chapter 12) emerged as fields of study. By 1997, Dr. Ritchie Shoemaker from Pokemoke, Maryland, began to write about toxins from infective agents in our environment as contributing to this greater world of illness, and he ultimately expanded this concept to include mold toxins and Lyme toxins as treatable disease components (Chapter 11). Dr. Jacob Teitelbaum (originally from Annapolis, Maryland), outlined this new model in his ground-breaking book on fibromyalgia and chronic fatigue, *From Fatigued to Fantastic!*

We will go over each of these ideas in much more detail, but the bigger picture, as it slowly emerged (so slowly as to go barely noticed at times), was that we were finding physical and biochemical deficiencies and imbalances as the root causes of our patients' suffering. When we correctly identified the imbalanced chemistry and treated it, often everything else got better, too. Patients who had been told they would have to live with feeling depressed, anxious, and fatigued were frequently cured and had no further need for the medications that had been prescribed for those conditions. We now had the beginnings of a whole new model for understanding and treating chronic illness, which allowed us to help many patients who had almost given up hope. That model continues to expand, and every year we acquire new information and tools to improve our abilities to support their healing process.

This growing body of information helped me understand that there was a whole world of healing out there, and that some of its techniques could help patients for whom my traditional medical skills were ineffective. Combining conventional medicine with this growing field of knowledge, which is now often called *holistic, alternative, complementary,* or *integrative medicine,* made a lot of sense. I could help significantly more patients than ever before, and just as importantly, I had new ways, or models, of how to understand their individual illnesses.

Over time, I started to work with more and more complicated patients. As a family physician, while I still dealt with sore throats and colds, my time was increasingly taken up by using the new concepts and ideas I had learned to help individuals heal when other methods had not been successful. As I solved certain problems, new patients came with even more complicated stories, and I needed more information, or tools, to be able to help them. This became an ebb and flow of my feeling inadequate, finding new fields to study, bringing this information back to my practice, helping some of the difficult patients whom I'd not adequately helped, and then getting even more complicated patients to treat, feeling inadequate, and again seeking new promising fields of study. Please understand that as we were able to help the vast majority of those who sought our assistance, these feelings were what drove us to continue to explore and learn even more.

I now have a large waiting list, and my staff and I have to work hard to prioritize our time so that we can take on the most difficult patients and refer those who are less ill to others.

This book is written with those "most difficult" patients in mind. In these pages, I would like to share my experience and knowledge with others, so those who have "fallen through the medical cracks" will know that there is hope for themselves and their families. It is my hope that this book will provide a starting point and direction so they can begin their journey of healing.

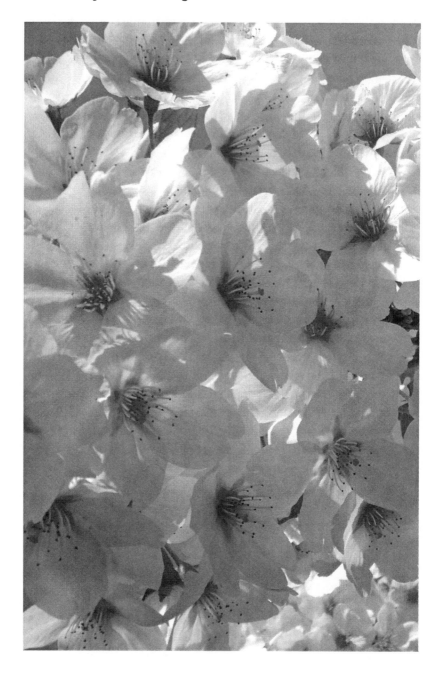

Chapter 2

The First Office Visit

It's All About the Diagnosis

*I*f you've picked up this book, then you're probably frustrated with your medical care and are convinced that something is wrong. Your team of doctors has exhausted its resources and can't seem to put a finger on the causes of your troubles. Somehow you get wind of a different approach and you want to check it out. How exactly does this work?

You start by contacting our office. Usually this is begun with a phone call, which is our preference since it is much more personal than an email or fax. You will talk to either our office manager or our nurse. Both are happy to answer your questions to be sure that you are not wasting your time with a visit; both are exceptional people in their caring and competence. Before you even get to our front door, we want you to know that we are concerned about your health and that we take your visit seriously. The office manager will get a detailed history that he can present to me for prioritization. We generally have a fair-sized waiting list, and over the years we have had to clarify our focus of the best use of my time. This means that those individuals who are interested in having me review their vitamin and supplement list are placed lower on the list, while those who are severely compromised and barely able to function go to the top of the list. Those who are referred by healthcare providers, particularly professionals known to us, go to the top of the list as well.

Our hope is that by the time we are ready to schedule you, you are ready for us as well. We ask, of course, that you bring as many medical records and reports as you can for review during or after the visit. Occasionally someone will express anger at me for my not reviewing those records beforehand, but I feel it's much more valuable for me to hear the whole story from my patients first, listening to how they express themselves and to the nuances of how illness has affected them. Then I will take a look at their records. Records are just pieces of paper and are not always correct, for they always reflect someone's opinions or biases, mine included. It is not unusual for patients to see their medical records, sometimes for the first time, and be astonished at how a healthcare provider saw their situation. "How could they have gotten that impression?" is a common response.

So you show up at our front door and walk inside. You will be greeted in a very friendly fashion and asked, of course, to complete some paperwork. The walls of my waiting room are covered with "joke photos," blown up pictures of me in various settings that I think are humorous. Most patients relax when they see those pictures, getting what I hope is the correct impression that we have a good sense of humor. A few are appalled by what they perceive to be my lack of professionalism, and this is a tip-off to the staff that these folks might need to lighten up a little. While we appreciate the seriousness of anyone's medical condition, life is difficult enough without the willingness to find some humor in it.

The nurse will take your vital signs and bring you back to see me. You are not undressed and left in a room for long periods of time. I try to be prompt, despite the nature of my work in which we can never know with certainty how long any visit will take. Being on time helps us to convey the message that your time is important, too.

We will spend the next hour or more going over your history in great detail, conducting a physical examination, and then putting together what I call a "smorgasbord." This is the part in which I try to summarize my understanding of your medical problem and lay out a wide variety of explanations and treatments. I will solicit your input in what you want to do, and in what order. If there is time left, and you have a specific area of pain or discomfort, I will try to fit in a preliminary treatment of osteopathic manipulation.

I would like to emphasize here, and repeat throughout this book, that *the central focus of each visit is to make a clear diagnosis.* I must identify with precision the cause(s) of my patients' symptoms in order to correctly treat those causes. Otherwise, I am simply shooting in the dark. Now, if you shoot in the dark, you might get lucky, but you can't count on that. It is obviously a better strategy for me to know what I'm doing with some clarity. Therefore, it is all about diagnosis. While it seems to me that this is such a simple concept, I fear that this process has been lost in the current practice of medicine. Before you leave our office, I want you to understand how we are going to get the information we need to make this clear diagnosis.

The most common feeling expressed by our patients at the first visit is surprise at our attentiveness to what they are saying and the thoroughness of the physical examination, which they have not had before.

After the history and physical exam, we will usually offer laboratory evaluation, which we draw at the initial visit, and a scheduled follow-up visit depending on what we've discovered. It is very important to me that you leave my office after your first visit filled with hope, and that you leave after every follow-up visit the same way. You see, I know you haven't had that experience before, and I hope to undo the negativity you have inadvertently received from previous healthcare providers, which has actually added another layer of interference with your healing process.

And so, we begin.

I thought it might be best to have some of my patients describe their experiences for you in their own words.

Katherine's Story

Doctors, Doctors, everywhere, but not one that can truly help me get well. So many meds, so many office visits and hospital stays. Eleven admits to the hospital in twelve months. Period. And I am still not well. The feeling I am on my own, of being misdiagnosed, going through the medical maze. Even feeling abandoned when a doctor or medical staff member is aloof, unkind, or impatient.

That was then; I needed to find a doctor who realized that because all people are different, we may not be able to be treated in the same way. I looked for that doctor a long time and found Dr. Nathan about twelve years ago. With much anxiety, I did not want to start all over again with another medical history and more medical reports. At times it takes hours. I made my appointment with Dr. Nathan and finally made it to the office, a very quiet room with overstuffed sofas. Not rows of fifty or more plastic and chrome hard chairs, and a crowded room . . . .

As I walk into the outer office, Kevin is there to great me, a very congenial young man. (Anyone under fifty is a young man!) He is both helpful and knowledgeable, with a light sense of humor to put you at ease. At most I wait ten minutes, not forty-five or more. I am ready for the treatment room. Neva says, "come in" in a very quiet but lilting voice. I feel I must be in the right place. Neva has a real gift of drawing blood and setting I.V.s. She has a very sensitive touch and is a truly capable assistant. I proceed to Dr. Nathan's room.

Doctor Nathan is a self-assured man with deep, penetrating eyes and a warm smile. I know now I am in the right place. (Okay, finally!)

"So what's happening with you?" he asks, although by the time he asks that question, he has a good idea. You spend about thirty minutes with Dr. Nathan, and understand what treatments you need to help get you well.

Now I am thinking, "That was easy. Ho!" There are lifestyle changes to be made. Some will take many months, maybe the rest of my life. "You try this until I see you again." If that doesn't work, Dr. Nathan always offers alternative methods, perhaps several. Sometimes when I think it is all too much for me, I am reminded of the sign on the door: No whining!

A very patient doctor, most times more of a teacher than a doctor, Dr. Nathan encourages you to learn, think, and read. Dr. Nathan has suggested so many books for me to read over the years, I have started the Neil J. Nathan Library, branch two.

We all need to take responsibility for our own illness and understand what is needed to get better. Dr. Nathan can't do that for us. He's here to help. Healing has to come from with-

in ourselves. Seeking knowledge, taking responsibility, and finding the right doctor may keep us from falling through the cracks.

It is very important to all of us that we make you comfortable and convey the message that healing is possible. Central to this process is the building of trust between us. Actually, you have no reason to trust me. Since the majority of my new patients have been through the mill and have spent a great deal of time and money getting frustrated, not feeling heard, and going nowhere, I realize that I have to work to create some kind of bond or working relationship that they have not experienced before. I do not take this for granted. Rather, I hope to review your information in enough detail that I can honestly offer you genuine hope that you *can* improve or heal.

Usually, your response to my suggestions over the first few months, based on your history and lab work, will convince you that healing is possible. Once that begins to occur, we have the first spark of trust, and I try to nurture that spark and build upon it. As improvement occurs, usually in fits and starts, we build slowly and carefully upon it, with the hope of each visit uncovering yet another clue that will allow us to understand your illness and treat it better. Sometimes patients, understandably motivated to move forward as soon as possible, push me to do everything at once. As eager as I am to do this, long years of experience have taught me that this will usually lead to confusion about what is working and what is not, and then we have to go back to square one again, losing ground. I hate losing ground, since it predisposes to the loss of trust and hope, both essential to what we are trying to build. So we go slowly, step-by-step, together, looking for the pieces of information that will move us in the direction of healing. This is a serious work-in-progress, and as long as both of us stay patient and focused, it is my experience that the vast majority of the time, good things will happen.

Heidi's Story

About six years ago, I began my search for a cure for the terrible pain I felt in my face. I was treated for several medical problems and tried many different medications to no avail. I was disappointed and frustrated. The neurologist who was treating me concluded that there was no cure and told me I would have to live with the facial pain the rest of my life. I felt despondent.

In desperation, I finally followed the suggestion of my friend and neighbor to call Dr. Nathan's office. I was told I would be put on a waiting list of thirty-seven people. I was worried I would have to wait a long time, but Dr. Nathan's administrative assistant, Kevin, told me to hang tough, and that eased my mind. About two weeks later, Kevin called to say there had been a cancellation. I was so eager to get relief from the pain that I rearranged my schedule so I could meet Dr. Nathan the next day.

My experience at Dr. Nathan's office has been very different from visits to other doctors. During our first meeting, Dr. Nathan conveyed a genuine concern for me and took an extensive history of the pain I had been having. I was pleased that he later shared this write-up with me because it made my relationship with him less mysterious. I believe our journey to get rid of the facial pain is a collaborative one. I like that Dr. Nathan gives me a thorough explanation of what he is going to do when he manipulates my head and that he asks if I understand what he is explaining.

When I first started cranial-sacral treatments, Dr. Nathan asked me if I felt scared, and he said that some people might consider these treatments to be "out there." I never felt scared, just desperate to be free from the pain and worried that this last attempt to do so might fail, just as the many medications I tried had failed.

❖

As Heidi's story reflects, many patients come to me as if I am the last resort, and, in fact, many use that phrase outright. It is part of my sense of humor to respond, "No, Las Vegas or Reno is the last resort." I want patients to understand that even if I cannot help them, or cure them, there is never a "last resort." I may not have the knowledge or skills to help them, but I am fairly sure that *someone* out there does, and with rare exceptions, one should not give up the hope that she will find that individual.

In the next section of this book, we will begin our journey into the exploration of exactly which biochemical imbalances our patient may have, and precisely what we can do about it. Although there will be some discussions of biochemistry in the upcoming material, I hope to explain this clearly enough that you will understand it without much struggle and will be able to build the picture in your mind of how we put all of this information together to create a healing plan.

Top Ten Things You *Won't* Find in Dr. Nathan's Office

1. Voice mail
2. Computerized scheduling
3. A crowded waiting room of patients annoyed at the ever-longer wait
4. A secretary who says "Hold, please." Click.
5. A physician more than twenty minutes late for your appointment
6. Endless discussions with a computer
7. Reams of computerized records thrown into a thick, unorganized chart
8. Staff members who refer to you as "the gallbladder in the treatment room"
9. Stacks of pre-printed referral forms
10. Charts with code words such as "Gomer, Crock, Whiner, Squirrel, or Turkey"

Top Ten Things You *Will* Find in Dr. Nathan's Office

1. Humor
2. Compassion
3. Skilled medical care
4. Staff that knows you in the office and in the grocery store as well
5. On-time service
6. Phone calls returned the same day
7. Quick response to health needs
8. The word "yes"
9. "Let me hear what you have to say"
10. Honesty

The "Big Six"

After I complete my initial history and physical evaluation of every new patient, the next step of our first visit is to sit down and talk about the most logical way for us to begin our evaluation and treatment program. Each patient is unique, and each story contains the clues that direct our attention to the treatments that are most likely to be helpful for that individual. But, as you might suspect, after awhile we begin to discern patterns that are common for many of our patients. After years of analyzing my patients' records, it became clear that some patterns, some testing, and some treatments were more frequently noted than others. So, over time, I evolved a somewhat simplified system to streamline this process.

To save my patients both time and money, we naturally started with the most commonly observed deficiencies, and then moved to the less common imbalances. This process was modified by attending to the details of my patients' stories. For example, if symptoms began following a severe infection, we might move evaluation and treatment of viral infections to a higher point on our wish list. If symptoms began following a dental procedure, we would evaluate mercury toxicity sooner, rather than later.

In general, however, I found that the majority of my patients had a group of imbalances that I came to call the "Big Six." New patients seemed to grasp this concept immediately, and for most of them the

"Big Six" were our starting point for evaluation and treatment.

By far the most common imbalance for my patients with complex, persistent illness is that of adrenal deficiency. While there are several types of adrenal imbalance, an inability to make an adequate amount of DHEA (the main hormone made by the adrenal gland) was present in well over 90 percent of my patients. This became job number one, so I call this "Step 1," and that will be our first chapter in this section. The next most common deficiency, noted in 80-85 percent of these patients, is that of magnesium, so that will be Step 2. Thyroid deficiency is statistically next most common and will be our Step 3. This is followed in frequency by sex hormone deficiencies, Step 4, and then by food allergy, Step 5, and the imbalance of our intestinal system will be Step 6.

The majority of my patients have not one but several of these imbalances, and we have found that fixing only one leads to only temporary improvement, followed by relapse. So I attempt to identify which of these apply to the patient sitting before me, and treat all of them. The response to treatment tells us what we have accomplished, and what we still need to do.

So if patients come back after treating all of these issues and tell me they are 60 percent better, this means that we have figured out 60 percent of what's wrong with them and still have 40 percent more to clarify. Then we move on to the next most common imbalances, which we will discuss in a later section.

I have discovered that this method simplifies the process of wading through complicated biological interactions. So, without further ado, let's get started by examining the six most common imbalances associated with chronic illness.

Chapter 3

Healing the Adrenal Glands

The Most Useful Test You've Never Heard Of: DHEA

When it comes to diagnosing, treating, and healing long-standing medical conditions, in my experience, the single most important and overlooked essential element is the functioning of the adrenal glands. In virtually all chronic medical conditions, the ability of the adrenal glands to respond appropriately to stress diminishes progressively as the stress of having that condition persists. Before we launch into this discussion, let's briefly examine the basic functions of these glands.

The adrenal glands are two small cone-shaped organs. One sits perched atop each kidney. They are essentially the "stress" glands of the body and are primarily responsible for how the body responds to all of the stressors placed upon it. These glands do not distinguish between the actual causes of stress, so physical stressors such as surgery, injury, childbirth, or chronic pain are just as much a strain on the adrenal glands as emotional or spiritual stressors. For the body, stress simply means the need to respond to change—any change. Even a positive one like getting a job promotion, starting a new and happy marriage, or winning the lottery would be experienced by the body as stressful, though our minds may be blissfully unaware of this. Incidents like these might feel wonderful, but they are nevertheless experienced by the body as changes, and a change in any form presents stress. It becomes clear, then, that merely feeling bad on a daily basis is more than sufficient to overtax and deplete the adrenal glands over time. For those of you who have been struggling with your health for a long time, studying adrenal function is our most logical starting point to seek out imbalances.

To oversimplify a bit, the adrenal glands make three major types of hormones: dehydroepiandrosterone (DHEA), mineralocorticoids, and cortisol. These hormones, in turn, make other hormones or affect how other hormones function. So these three hormones are really important to the metabolism of the body. Let's discuss these three hormonal areas in detail.

Dehydroepiandrosterone (DHEA)

The largest amount of hormone produced by the adrenals comes in the form of DHEA, which stands for *dehydroepiandrosterone*. As with many medical chemical names, this is quite a mouthful, so we'll stick with its abbreviation, DHEA. The good news is that DHEA levels are relatively easy to measure with a simple, readily available blood test. And a measured DHEA deficiency is even easier to treat, using pure supplements that you can purchase from any natural food store.

From the outset of our discussion, I would like to emphasize that if I had only one lab test and treatment available to me to provide help for my chronically ill patients, that would be DHEA. It is, to my mind, the most useful test I have.

Let's talk about DHEA for a bit so we can understand the nature and value of this, one of our most important natural hormones. DHEA is a precursor for a host of other hormones, the best-known including estrogen and testosterone. Most of those other hormones have long chemical names which are difficult to pronounce, and a detailed discussion of this chemistry is far beyond the scope of this book. However, it can simply be said that in order for us to remain in balance as we wrestle with stress, we have to centrally produce a wide array of hormones that allow us to deal with stress properly. If we can't, we lose the ability to cope with stress adequately, not only psychologically, but also physically.

This would seem to be a tremendously important factor to illness, but for reasons that I cannot understand, this information has not received much attention from the medical profession. It is not unusual for me to see patients who have been researching their symptoms, and many of them, without benefit of a medical degree, have realized that they are probably depleted in adrenal hormones. When they present this idea to their primary care providers, almost all report that this suggestion falls on deaf ears. When we measure their DHEA levels, they are universally low, and our patients usually remark, "Ah, I'm not surprised." It is extremely rare for me to see a patient whose DHEA level has been measured by her primary care physician. Why? I suspect that many physicians have come to believe that the only possible manifestation of adrenal deficiency is in the form called *Addison's disease.* This is a rare condition in which the adrenal glands have been permanently and severely damaged, and those patients will require adrenal hormone replacement for the rest of their lives, usually provided by specialists in endocrinology. Somehow, conventional medicine has yet to embrace the concept that the adrenal glands can be temporarily weakened—not always permanently damaged—and can be successfully treated.

The bottom line here is that we need an adequate supply of DHEA to be able to make our adrenal hormones. When we began our discussion of the adrenal glands in this chapter, we focused on stress in all forms. As any stress persists, whether physical or emotional, the adrenal glands slowly lose their ability to keep up with those hormonal demands and start to become depleted. In my experience, the most common deficiency in most chronic illness is this deficiency of DHEA. Well over 90 percent of my patients with fibromyalgia and chronic fatigue are deficient in this hormone, often to a profound degree. In fact, since almost any chronic condition is clearly associated with significant stress, we find a deficiency of DHEA in almost all of our patients. Those patients who have been receiving significant doses of synthetic cortisone materials like prednisone or prednisolone on a regular basis can be virtually guaranteed that their levels of DHEA will be extremely low, as those medications turn off and inhibit normal adrenal function.

Symptoms of DHEA Deficiency

Essentially, a deficiency of DHEA causes fatigue, fatigue, and more fatigue. What's more, it also creates a slew of other symptoms:

- Tiredness
- Exhaustion
- "I just don't feel like myself"
- Cognitive Impairment (brain fog)
- Decreased Libido
- Recurrent Infections
- Depression

Since the majority of my patients have been sick for quite some time before their initial visit to me, fatigue is a problem for almost every one of them. One of my questions at our first interview is to ask the patient to rate his energy level on a scale of zero to ten, where "ten" means a full tank of gas, and "zero" means running on empty. If a patient's response is "eight or nine," that's fairly normal. But if the response is "two or three," which is quite common, then I have a nice, almost quantitative estimate of the extent of his fatigue, which of course is subjective. I find this initial number useful as a baseline by which to measure the patient's progress as we move along in treatment.

Testing and Evaluating DHEA Levels

Measuring DHEA is easy. It can be measured in two different forms. One of them is unconjucated or "plain" DHEA, and the other is DHEA-S, which is bound to sulfate. I prefer measuring the unconjugated form because I believe it to be the most accurate measurement. Other physicians prefer to evaluate DHEA-S, which is the storage form of the hormone. Either way, a simple blood test can be used to learn quickly where patients stand in terms of their DHEA levels.

Interpreting these test results, however, requires a little more work and a little more information. First of all, the normal values for DHEA from the laboratory I use are 130-980 (ng/dL) for women and 180-1250 (ng/dL) for men. Clearly these numbers represent a huge range, and many physicians are not aware that, unlike other tests, the reason for this large spread is that these values are *age-based*. That is, 130 would be a normal level for a ninety-year-old woman, while 980 would be normal for a teenage girl. The same is true for men: 180 is normal for a ninety-year-old, and 1250 would be normal for a teenager. Once we understand this relationship—the fact that the age of the patient and her DHEA value are directly correlated—we can then extrapolate the test results, by age, to find out what the number means.

Let's say one of my fifty-year-old male patients has a level of 200. A quick glance at his lab report would define this as a normal level (and the computer obligingly places it there). If these reports are carelessly evaluated, some physicians could be led astray into thinking that value of 200 was normal. But it's not. According to the clearly established age-level relationship, a fifty-year-old male should be about halfway between 180 and 1250, or roughly 600-700. All of a sudden that 200 looks awfully low, which it is. In fact, it's almost a third of what it should be, and it is likely that providing DHEA supplementation will make a big difference for this individual in his healing process.

You can see from the wide "normal" values for DHEA that it is an excellent example of a hormone whose levels decline profoundly as we get older. Some researchers have even suggested that, to a certain extent, aging may be reversed by keeping DHEA levels close to optimal, although what that optimal level might be is not currently clear. This concept has led some to call it the "fountain of youth hormone." I'm certainly not prepared to go that far, but I do know that measuring and treating this hormone deficiency is an excellent first step in beginning to bring a weakened physiology back to a healthy and sustainable state.

Treatment of DHEA Deficiency

Just as diagnosing DHEA deficiency is a relatively simple process, so too are treatment and supplementation. Pharmaceutical grade (high quality) DHEA can be purchased from any natural food store, and it is usually taken orally, in capsule form, once a day, usually in the morning. However, the dosage that patients need depends on the measured level of the hormone. I strongly discourage those of you who suspect a deficiency of DHEA from treating yourself. As with any hormonal treatment, guidance from an experienced clinician is important. Sometimes, when I use the word "hormone," patients immediately jump to the idea of female hormones, like estrogen, and they lump all these hormones together in their minds. This assumption makes them leery of taking anything "hormonal." It is important for us to realize that we have hundreds of hormones circulating through our body at all times, and the fears currently associated with estrogen usage (see Chapter 6) do not apply to all hormones equally. DHEA is a very different hormone than estrogen, and as you will see, it has very few side effects. It is safe enough that the FDA allows it to be sold without prescription in health food stores. But although DHEA is admittedly a much safer hormone than most, you still don't want to take any hormonal substance if you don't know for sure your body needs it. And as we've seen, measuring it is so easy.

So, while they are quite uncommon, there can be a few minor side effects from using DHEA. In my experience, about 5 to 10 percent of women (rarely men) will break out in facial acne from its use, and if this happens the treatment must be either discontinued or the dose decreased. Some women will also complain of an increased growth of facial hair. Because the DHEA supplements improve energy, they may interfere with sleep if taken too late in the day. I recommend that the full dose always be taken in the morning.

It is also important to note that DHEA must not be taken by patients who have been diagnosed with breast, ovarian, or prostate cancer. As we noted earlier, to a minor extent, DHEA is converted by the body into estrogen and testosterone, and tumors that are hormonally sensitive could potentially grow in the presence of DHEA. This information has unfortunately confused some patients into thinking that DHEA may cause cancer. This is not the case; in fact, the opposite is true. Research indicates that DHEA deficiency weakens the immune system (hence an increased tendency to recurrent infections). Thus, it is more likely that a patient with a measured low level of DHEA would actually improve his or her immune function and prevent cancer by taking the supplement. Understanding the difference here is vital: DHEA affects only existing tumors and does not produce new ones.

Having said all of this about side effects, readers should understand that the vast majority of patients can take DHEA without experiencing any of them. It has far fewer side effects than aspirin.

As I will repeat throughout this book, the single most important thing to look at is how each individual patient responds to the treatment we are providing. If taking DHEA leads to improvement, it is clearly useful. If not, we have to question its usefulness, even if the blood tests are low. Note that it takes approximately two to six weeks to see improvement both clinically and in DHEA levels once daily supplementation has started. If no improvement occurs, we may need to recheck the blood level at six to eight weeks to be sure the hormone is being absorbed and utilized properly by the body. Once a patient has responded well, she usually can discontinue taking DHEA after about a year and not need supplementation again.

My office has measured and treated more than 5,000 patients with DHEA deficiency over the past twenty years. The response to treatment is so gratifying that I cannot think of a single test that has been more useful in helping to heal all forms of chronic illness. Most patients who test low for DHEA will indeed respond to treatment with improvement ranging from mild to dramatic. Hence, this little measurement really forms the cornerstone of the testing process and the beginning of our looking for treatable biochemical deficiencies that will begin the healing process.

Travis's Story

Travis was thirty-five years old when he came to see me after experiencing some unusual complications, stemming from what he thought was just a simple injury. He had jumped over a fence and had fallen awkwardly onto a short, rock wall, landing on his left lower rib cage. He was incredibly sore for several days but didn't think much of it until a rather violent sneeze one week later sent him into paroxysms of pain. Later that night, he collapsed while getting up to go to the bathroom. Sweaty and unable to breathe, Travis was taken by ambulance to the emergency room, where he collapsed again, suffering a brief loss of consciousness, rapid pulse, and low blood pressure. For a short time he was unable to breathe. His doctors thought this was probably caused by a pulmonary embolus (a blood clot in the pulmonary artery), and he was immediately admitted to the hospital and treated for the presumed embolus. All of this treatment was completely appropriate, even though testing proved inconclusive, which is not unusual for this condition.

Over the next several weeks, Travis developed swelling in

both legs, and his doctors documented deep vein thromboses (blood clots) in both legs, with a greater number on his right side than his left. These were aggressively and properly treated with heparin, a blood thinning medication, which eventually eliminated the blood clots. But then Travis started to develop a swelling of the lymph nodes in his groin and a persistent soreness and occasional catches in the muscles of his chest wall. He underwent a biopsy of his lymph nodes to be sure that this was not cancer. It wasn't.

Since his original injury four months previously, he had become overwhelmingly fatigued. Prior to his injury, he had been a very energetic young man who not only held down a full-time job, but also worked long extra hours doing landscaping work. He was proud of the fact that he had been able to work these long hours for many years, with no loss in vitality. But now, for the first time in his life, he was barely able to manage his primary job. Actually, he had to take several months off, and was now only able to work six hours a day. He was so frustrated and upset by his inability to function as he once had, that he couldn't even think about doing his landscaping work. He had been so proud of his physical strength, and now it was gone. He was worried about this bizarre turn of events following a seemingly minor injury and was starting to think, "What will happen to me next?" Now, in addition to feeling physically weak, with steady pain across his lower left rib cage, he was frightened as well.

At his first visit with me, Travis was clearly confused and afraid. He could not see how he had become so profoundly weakened in just a few months from this seemingly trivial injury. From my perspective, his physicians had done a good job of treating his initial injuries and their sequelae (the blood clots), but they had not taken the time to explain to Travis the logical sequence in which all of these events had occurred. Since his fear was prominent, my first task was to clarify this sequence for him and his family. After I explained to him that the injury had set off a delayed blood clot—which in turn had made him dizzy and faint and required the hospital care he had received—and that the lymph nodes in his groin were just the normal result of healing the blood clots, Travis could begin to see this chain of events as less mysterious. I then explained how these physical stressors to his body had weakened his adrenal glands, and that by measuring his DHEA and treating it, he could likely recover his health.

When we measured Travis's DHEA, it turned out to be 160 ng/dL. A normal level for his age would be closer to 800. I started him on 50 mg of DHEA each morning, and treated his rib cage with osteopathic manipulation (see Chapter 17). Within two weeks he was back in the office with a smile on his face. He was back at work full-time again, and he was no longer collapsing on the couch after work. His rib cage pain was gone. He had resumed his extra landscaping work and was handling it well, and was now feeling like himself again. He was astonished at the rapidity of this energetic turn around. I was not as surprised as he, as I have seen this response so frequently that I've come to take it as a matter of course.

While Travis's recovery is clearly impressive and a bit atypical since it occurred faster than usual, it illustrates how important and valuable looking for DHEA deficiency can be. As you read through my patients' stories in this book, you will notice that most of them responded well to DHEA as a part of their treatments.

Karen's Story

Karen was a forty-year-old woman who came to my office with a long history of thyroid problems. Several years previously, she had been diagnosed as having fibromyalgia and chronic fatigue. She noted that on a bad day she would lie in bed all day and move very little, and on a good day she would get up and try to do things, and that really exhausted her. Her body throbbed and her muscles were in constant pain. When she woke up in the morning, it was like she'd been "beaten with a baseball bat all night." It would usually take her un-

til noon to get dressed and start moving. She reported that she couldn't handle stress; it wiped her out. She was usually irritable. Routine blood tests, including thyroid tests, were normal. Antidepressants taken over a ten-year period of time were of little to no benefit. She described her energy level as "between zero and two," on a scale of ten. Despite excessive sleep, she was completely unrefreshed when she awoke. She had been researching her own problem and decided she had Wilson's syndrome (which we will describe in Chapter 5).

We started by measuring Karen's DHEA level, which came back at 224 ng/dL. (A normal level for her age would be about 600.) Because of her low measured level of DHEA, we started her on 50 mg supplements each morning. When I saw her for a follow-up consultation two months later, she reported that she was doing extremely well and estimated that she was about "85 percent better." She had only minor joint pains now, which mostly occurred when she overworked herself. Her overall mood had also improved dramatically. We elected to see if just continuing this treatment with no additional elements would be sufficient to produce complete resolution of her symptoms, and it was.

So Karen is yet another example of the remarkable improvement that is possible with the simple addition of DHEA. While most of my patients are quite a bit more complicated than Karen, it is most gratifying to see someone get her life back so quickly.

However, if patients do respond well to supplementation with DHEA, but not completely, we may have to look a little deeper into their adrenal function to determine if the problem is beyond a simple DHEA deficiency.

Mineralocorticoids

A second hormonal function of the adrenal gland is its assistance in helping to regulate blood pressure. The adrenals make what are called *mineralocorticoids*, a group of hormones that help to raise the blood pressure when it is low. Most of us are aware that *high* blood pressure is not a good thing, but it is not as well known that *low* blood pressure isn't good for us either. In essence, your blood pressure is very similar to the water pressure in your home. If your water pressure is too low and you try to take a shower, the water will simply trickle out of the shower head because there isn't enough pressure to push it out of the spout. Low blood pressure is just the same: you aren't pumping enough blood through your body to provide adequate circulation, and this can lead to fatigue and weakness.

A particular symptom that can tip us off to the presence of low blood pressure is that of dizziness or lightheadedness when standing up or changing position abruptly. The technical medical name for this condition is orthostatic hypotension. This symptom can be formally diagnosed by a tilt-table testing procedure, originally described by researchers at Johns Hopkins in the mid-nineties. However, in my experience, it isn't necessary to do this expensive testing to confirm the diagnosis. When we see a patient with consistently low blood pressures, and those pressures drop even further on standing up, we can make a presumptive diagnosis and work with our patient empirically. This means that we can simply provide treatment for the unusually low blood pressure, presuming the presence of a mineralocorticoid deficiency, and see how our patient responds. We have the choice of two medications that specifically improve mineralocorticoid production: Florinef and Midodrine. How each individual patient responds to this treatment is our key as to whether or not we're on the right path to healing.

When I mention this treatment to some patients, they are frightened by the possibility that it will raise their blood pressure to dangerous levels. I can assure you that this isn't possible. The most I've seen these medications elevate blood pressure is about ten points for both upper (systolic) and lower (diastolic) blood pressure readings. This means that a pressure of 90/60 won't go much higher than 100/70. However, that small rise in pressure may make all the difference in the world to a fatigued patient, and it certainly adds another dimension to our treatment. Please keep in mind that this does not mean that all patients with low blood pressures need this type of treatment. For the majority of patients who are found to have low blood pressures, those pressures are normal. Only those with chronic fatigue and a tendency to get dizzy or lightheaded when they stand up suddenly should even consider the possibility of taking these medications and, again, only under clinical supervision. In fact, Florinef and Midodrine are available only by prescription.

When we do use these medications, it is rare for a patient to need them for more than a few months. It's almost as if the body occasionally seems to forget how to properly make the hormones it needs, and by this gentle medicinal reminder, given for brief periods of time, it gets back on track.

Cortisol

The third main form of adrenal deficiency is that of the hormone *cortisol*, which is essential to a wide variety of healthy functions. When cortisol is not made in adequate amounts by the body, especially in response to stress, we see fatigue, exhaustion, allergies, hirsutism (abnormal hair growth), and a tendency towards miscarriage for women who are pregnant. But, as I've been emphasizing throughout this chapter, cortisol regulates the ability of the body to deal with stress of any kind.

Some of the most extensive research in this area was done by William M. Jeffries, M.D., whose many papers and books on the subject are summarized in his seminal book, *Safe Uses of Cortisol*. Jeffries emphasizes that there is a huge difference between small physiological doses of natural cortisol and large doses of synthetic cortisones, like prednisone. A physiological dose of a hormone is the amount of hormone that the body would naturally manufacture if it is able to do so. Please note the wording difference between *cortisol* and *cortisone*, because, although these words are very similar, we are talking about different substances. Both cortisol and cortisone are the natural hormones made by the adrenal glands. Confusion about these words comes about because we generally refer to the *synthetic* materials that are similar to the natural adrenal materials as "cortisone" also. Since most of my patients are aware of the toxic effects produced by long-term use of synthetic cortisone, they are often reluctant to even consider taking small doses of cortisol, until we explain the enormous differences between the natural and synthetic materials. The essence of Jeffries' research is that tiny amounts of cortisol may be restorative to the body when we have identified cortisol deficiency, as opposed to the large doses of synthetic cortisone that are traditionally used in a wide variety of medical conditions and carry a much greater risk of toxicity.

In treatment, we begin by measuring the cortisol deficiency of the patient so that we know what we're looking at. The test we use is called a *cortrosyn stimulation test,* a standard analysis used in conventional endocrinology for this exact purpose. Natural cortisol is produced while we sleep, in what is described as a circadian rhythm. Our blood levels of cortisol peak at about 8 a.m. and slowly drop throughout the day, in this natural cycle. Thus, it is standard for us to measure the patient's baseline cortisol at 8 a.m. and then provide an injection of cortrosyn, a pituitary stimulant that should, if the adrenal gland is working properly, triple the baseline level of cortisone. If the adrenal gland cannot respond appropriately to this natural stimulation, which mimics exactly how the adrenal gland should respond to a natural stressor, then we know we are dealing with a cortisol deficiency. Dr. Jeffries aptly named this *mild adrenal insufficiency* to distinguish it from the much more severe deficiency known as Addison's disease, which we have already mentioned. We can treat these mild cases of deficiency by providing small doses of cortisone acetate, also known as Cortef, or hydrocortisone acetate, which is just a little bit stronger than Cortef. Dr. Jeffries has found that as long as we keep the dose of Cortef at less than 40 mg daily, there are virtually no side effects, even with prolonged administration of this hormone for up to forty-five years. As this is a hormonal medication, it can only be provided by a physician, preferably one trained in its use.

Once again, patient response is the key. If the patient improves from cortisol treatment, with a significant decrease in fatigue, we have identified yet another component of his illness. If not, even with abnormally low laboratory testing results, we must go back to the drawing board.

We as medical professionals must become more attentive to how our patients respond to different treatments. The truth of the treatment is in its success, or lack thereof, for each individual patient. With both the mineralocorticoid and natural cortisol treatments, the nice thing is that once patients have responded, they don't need to take these medications forever.

As mentioned previously, the majority of patients who take the mineralocorticoids find that after two to three months, they have restimulated their adrenals into better working order, and their blood pressure has normalized and stays that way. For hydrocortisone, usually after a year or two, the adrenal is back up and running and the medication can be discontinued forever. Recall that the same is true for DHEA: most patients placed on it can discontinue it after about a year.

What we appear to be doing with this approach is restoring adrenal function to normal. And that seems to be a really good thing for our fatigued and chronically ill patients, as they start back on the road to health.

Carla's Story

Carla was forty-eight when she came to see me, hoping that I could help cure her pain. She was on a slew of medications and had become really concerned about their possible long-term side effects. She also wanted to know why she stayed so tired and exhausted all the time—all she wanted was "more spunk."

Carla reported that, except for some minor aches and pains, she had been well until six years previously, when she received a flu shot. Two days later she developed a severe pain that radiated from her left shoulder at the site of her vaccination and up into her neck and shoulder. After the initial onset of pain, she continued to have pain between her shoulder blades and developed additional pain across her lower back and hips. Some days were worse than others. She had seen multiple physicians and chiropractors and she had been given many diagnoses, including fibromyalgia, osteoarthritis, a bulged disc in her neck, and even osteoporosis. She rated her energy as "five" on a scale of zero to ten. If she expected to get any sleep, she had to take Flexeril (a muscle relaxant), and if she expected to function at all, she needed to take various pain and anti-inflammatory medications.

I completed a DHEA blood test on Carla and discovered that she was at less than half of the normal amount for her age. Her initial measurement read 235 ng/dL, but for her age it should have been about 500. So I started her on 25 mg of DHEA each morning. I discovered that she had low levels of estrogen and progesterone as well, so I provided her with bio-

identical hormones (see Chapter 6). I also found overgrowth of the yeast Candida in a stool culture, which we treated (see Chapter 8). On this healing regimen, Carla improved somewhat over a period of four months. In addition to these supplements, I specifically treated her hip, back, neck, and shoulders with osteopathic manipulations and injections (see Chapter 17). As is typical for many of these patients, Carla noted that she got a little better after each treatment we added. Her path to healing was to be constructed of small stepping stones. She was better now by her own estimate of "30 to 40 percent." But she was still not completely well.

As we dug deeper to find the missing pieces of Carla's puzzling illness, I realized that her blood pressures were consistently low, measuring 94/60 on two consecutive visits, and she did get dizzy sometimes when standing up too quickly. So I offered her a trial of Florinef, 0.1 mg each morning. At the same time, I conducted a Cortrosyn stimulation test on Carla, which showed a baseline level of cortisol at 14.7 mcg/dL. It increased to only 29.1 mcg/dL thirty minutes following her injection of Cortrosyn. For her, an appropriate response to the Cortrosyn should have reached triple the original 14.7 mcg/dL, or 44.1 mcg/dL, whereas we measured it at only 29.1. Over several months, we slowly increased her dose of oral Cortef until it reached 30 mg daily. She noted significant improvement in her energy and well-being as we slowly increased her dose. As she had observed, she had an initial improvement of about 30 to 40 percent with our first treatments, and now reported that she was an additional 30 percent better with our additional adrenal treatments using Cortef and Florinef. Her blood pressure came up to more normal levels, her dizziness cleared, and I was able to discontinue the Florinef treatments after just three months. She slowly continued to improve on her treatment program and now considers herself "almost cured."

Carla's story is evidence that identifying and treating these adrenal deficiencies can lead to improvements, even in those who have been ill for years. Further improvements for Carla occurred when we discovered and treated her mold toxicity (see Chapter 11) and methylation imbalances (see Chapter 14), but those are stories that we will tell as this book unfolds.

Thanks for staying with me. I know that some of this information is highly technical, but I hope that you can begin to understand that, although this chemistry may be complicated, the essence of it is actually quite simple: Stress depletes adrenal function, but the good news is that we can identify, measure, and treat these imbalances to begin the process of healing.

Further Reading

Jeffries, William M. *Safe Uses of Cortisol*. 2nd ed. Springfield, IL: Charles C. Thomas, 1996.

Shealy, C. N. *DHEA: The Youth and Health Hormone*. New Canaan, CT: Keats, 1996.

Chapter 4

Magnesium Deficiency

The Little Mineral That Could

*T*he second most common deficiency often missed in patients who have chronic illnesses is that of magnesium. Most of us have heard a lot about calcium, especially with recent concerns about osteoporosis in women, and while calcium intake is stressed, magnesium gets little attention. Calcium and magnesium are a little like two sides of a coin: it is vitally important that they be in balance within the body. All of the cells in our bodies are bathed in calcium and filled inside with magnesium. The body likes it that way—it has elaborate safeguards in place to make certain that magnesium stays inside its cells, and that calcium stays outside. In simplistic terms, you might think of the aging process as the slow leakage of calcium into the cells, which make them more rigid and less responsive.

For reasons which have not yet been clarified, most chronic disease processes cause magnesium to leak out of the cells and to be eliminated from the body by the kidneys. I've found that in 90 percent of my chronic-pain patients and in 80 percent of my patients experiencing depression, chronic fatigue, and fibromyalgia, magnesium is depleted. In some patients, this depletion is mild; in others, profound.

Symptoms of Deficiency

Since magnesium is a critical mineral in all muscle and nerve functions, when our bodies are deficient in it, we see fatigue, depression, malaise, muscle cramps and pain, and difficulties with focus, memory and concentration. In addition, magnesium is a critical co-factor in hundreds of chemical reactions in the body, so when we have an insufficient amount of this little mineral, we may experience multiple symptoms and organ difficulties. The following list illustrates some of the major symptoms of magnesium deficiency:

- Fatigue, exhaustion, tiredness
- Muscle cramps, spasm, and pain
- Muscle weakness
- Manual treatments (chiropractic, physical therapy, manipulation) do not "hold" or last more than a few hours
- Depression
- Cardiac arrhythmias (irregular heartbeats or palpitations)
- Cognitive impairment (difficulty with focus, memory or concentration)
- Insomnia

Testing and Evaluating

So if magnesium is this important, why don't more physicians measure and treat it? First of all, most physicians don't know *how* to measure it accurately. When magnesium is measured by most physicians, usually for alcoholics and cardiac patients who commonly exhibit magnesium deficiency, it is usually measured by a blood test. We pointed out that magnesium is usually found inside of cells and not in the blood stream. The body thinks that magnesium is so important that it will do everything in its power to keep the blood levels of magnesium at a constant level. To do so, if it is deficient, the body will literally pull magnesium out of cells to keep blood levels normal. Thus, you could have a perfectly normal blood test result and still have really low magnesium levels inside your cells.

The golden standard for accurately measuring magnesium levels is called the Magnesium Challenge Test, in which levels are measured in the urine before and after the administration of magnesium supplementation. This test is rather cumbersome to perform, and I have found that a much simpler test is just as accurate: the *intracellular* measurement.

This is not a blood test, but a scraping of cells from under the tongue, a procedure my patients fondly call a "pap smear of the tongue." The scraped cells are placed on a glass slide and sent to a lab where the levels of intracellular magnesium can be ascertained. I have personally found this to be the most accurate test for measuring this critical mineral and it is often abnormal, even when the blood test shows otherwise; hence, it is far more useful in making our diagnosis.

Normal levels for intracellular magnesium are defined as 33.9-41.9 mEq/L. A mild deficiency corresponds to 33.0-33.9 mEq/L, a moderate deficiency is 31.0-33.0 mEq/L, and a severe deficiency is lower than 31.0 mEq/L. Making these distinctions is important, because when the body is running low on magnesium, it paradoxically loses the ability to absorb magnesium properly from the intestines. Logic would suggest that if you have a really low magnesium level by measurement, you could just take more by mouth to make up the difference. Sorry, but this strategy won't work, and I will tell you why.

Treatment

Our bodies have a limited capacity to absorb magnesium from the intestines. When that capacity is exceeded, we get the one symptom that too much magnesium produces: diarrhea. In fact, if you think about it, milk of magnesia and magnesium citrate are commonly used as laxatives, taking advantage of that side effect. However, while useful for treating constipation (for brief periods of time), oral magnesium supplementation works on the bowel by increasing transit time, a fancy way of saying that everything in your intestines moves through the system much faster. When this occurs, it doesn't allow the body enough time to digest and absorb food, nutrients, supplements, and minerals—it all moves through the body too quickly. So simply taking lots of magnesium orally will not work to accommodate deficiency.

Therefore, for severe or moderate deficiencies, we find it necessary to provide magnesium intravenously. Doing this gives the mineral the advantage of bypassing the intestines, going straight into the body and providing a larger amount for the body than it would obtain by simply ingesting it. A series of these intravenous treatments is often profoundly helpful in chronically ill patients. I use a version of what is called the Myers' cocktail, named after the physician in Baltimore who developed it. This cocktail includes magnesium, calcium, and vitamins C and B-12. The number of intravenous treatments provided depends on the level of magnesium depletion noted on the test. However, sometimes even in the face of normal tests, patients respond really well to these treatments. There are virtually no side effects of the intravenous magnesium. While the original Myers' cocktail was often given by "push," meaning it went right into the vein, I find it much gentler to give this infusion over forty-five minutes to an hour. If given too quickly, patients may notice flushing or headache, which resolve quickly as the drip is slowed.

So should all chronically ill patients take magnesium? Probably. Note, however, that all magnesium formulas are not created equal. Most magnesium that you buy over the counter is entirely or mostly composed of magnesium oxide because it is inexpensive to manufacture. Unfortunately, the oxide form of magnesium is not well absorbed by the body. Only 10 percent of the magnesium in this form is actually absorbed. For other forms of magnesium, particularly the chelated forms, up to 50 percent can be absorbed by the body. I prefer magnesium taurate, which is magnesium attached to taurine (an amino acid commonly depleted by stress), thus giving my patients two nutrients for the price of one. Some manufacturers have suggested that colloidal minerals are even easier for the body to absorb orally, but to my knowledge there is no evidence to substantiate that claim.

Jim's Story

While I have promised the majority of my patients that their real names will not be used in these vignettes, in a few instances, I've been given permission to provide the true name.

I have known my osteopathic mentor and friend, Jim Jealous, D.O., for over thirty years. He has always seemed in robust health, as we have hiked and snow-shoed over the White Mountains of New Hampshire, where he lives. So it came as quite a surprise when he called me a number of years ago to describe his recent health changes. Under significant stress, he had developed heart palpitations with cardiac arrhythmias, accompanied by fatigue and insomnia, elevated blood pressure, and an overall sense of feeling poorly. He reported severe muscle spasms as he slept, especially when he assumed certain postures. When he called, he had just been released from his local hospital, and despite their best efforts, he was no better. These symptoms were completely new for Jim, and he was worried that with the use of the medications prescribed for him, he was not addressing the real causes of his symptoms. So he flew out to see me.

With a little testing, it became immediately clear that he was working with a profound magnesium deficiency, which we measured at 31.6 mEq/L (normal levels are 33.9-41.0 mEq/L). This had in turn caused significant calcium depletion as well. Jim's calcium level was 8.0 mg/dL (normal levels are 8.5-10.5 mg/dL). Amazingly, his physicians had not measured either of these, despite his cardiac symptoms, which included atrial fibrillation and elevated blood pressure!

I provided Jim with intravenous magnesium, calcium, and manganese for several days in a row and made arrangements for him to continue this treatment when he returned home. However, he was delighted to report that after his first infusion he was able to sleep through the night for the first time in eight months. By the time he left our office, he was markedly better. Within just a few weeks, Jim's fatigue had lifted, along with his overall sense of poor health. His arrhythmias had virtually disappeared, and his blood pressure had come down to a much safer, controlled level. As he continued to receive magnesium treatments, he returned to his former state of excellent health.

Jim's story is an excellent example of how replacing a single vital nutrient can profoundly and rapidly improve someone's health.

❖

Further Reading

Gaby, Alan. "Intravenous Nutrient Therapy: The Myers' Cocktail."
Alternative Medicine Review 7.5 (2002): 389–403.

"Intracellular Tissue Analysis." *Exatest.com*. Intracellular Diagnostics,
Inc. 2009. Web. 15 Nov. 2009. *(IntraCellular Diagnostics is
the laboratory I use for most of my magnesium testing. Their
Web site provides an extensive bibliography of downloadable
medical papers on magnesium deficiency.)*

Seelig, Mildred. "Review and Hypothesis: Might Patients with the
Chronic Fatigue Syndrome have Latent Tetany of Magnesium
Deficiency?" *Journal of Chronic Fatigue Syndrome* 4.2 (1998):
77–108.

Chapter 5

Thyroid Function

If It Looks Like a Duck, Quacks Like a Duck, and Waddles Like a Duck, It Just Might Be . . .

*A*nother common imbalance often overlooked in chronically ill patients is that of thyroid deficiency. This discussion will reflect another controversial concept in our understanding of the chemistry of chronic illness. Conventional medicine has traditionally only acknowledged one form of thyroid deficiency, technically referred to as *hypothyroidism,* from the prefix *hypo* meaning *low.* This accepted form of thyroid deficiency reflects damage to the thyroid gland, resulting in the inability of the thyroid to produce sufficient hormone. This results in a condition that is easily diagnosed with blood tests and treated with thyroid hormone replacement. All physicians would agree with the truth of this description.

However, there is a growing awareness among some physicians that this somewhat rigid definition of thyroid deficiency does not take into account another form of hypothyroidism, which is actually not uncommon. Patients often come to my office having researched their own symptoms and are convinced that their thyroid needs treatment, but they've been told on the basis of repeated thyroid blood tests that their thyroid is normal and cannot be a part of their illness. I often find that they are correct, and that we need to evaluate and treat this gland in order to move toward healing.

The thyroid gland is a butterfly-shaped organ that gently wraps around the front of your neck. On the inside, the gland is hard at work trying to balance your metabolism. Because the essence of thyroid function is about the regulation of metabolism, deficiencies would naturally create a sluggish chemistry that would affect every part of the body. It should not come as a surprise, therefore, that low levels of thyroid hormones are associated with a variety of symptoms:

- Fatigue
- Constipation
- Temperature dysregulation (LOW)
- Hair loss (especially the lateral third of the eyebrow)
- Dry skin
- Menstrual abnormalities
- Cognitive impairment (difficulties with focus, memory, concentration and depression)

The essence lies in the phrase *sluggish metabolism*; every chemical reaction in the body is slower. As I have mentioned, countless patients who feel ill have read about this and felt that they might have a thyroid problem, often to be told by their physicians on the sole basis of blood tests that they do not. How can that be? The problem here, I suspect, is that there are several types of thyroid deficiency, and that the blood tests available to us as physicians only measure *one* of them.

Wilson's Syndrome

I would like to emphasize that virtually all physicians agree that if indeed the thyroid gland is clearly and permanently damaged by radiation, surgery, or autoimmune disease (the most common type being *Hashimoto's thyroiditis*), then standard blood tests would reflect this and show definitively who actually needs treatment. On this we all agree, and such patients diagnosed with this type of irreparable damage should receive thyroid hormone treatments, usually for their entire lifetime.

What we don't all agree upon is the existence of another form of thyroid deficiency, one that doesn't show up on blood tests but still reflects a genuine need for thyroid hormone replacement. This deficiency is sometimes referred to as *Wilson's syndrome*, which must be distinguished from a rare copper-excess condition called *Wilson's dis-*

ease. Research in this area first received attention in the 1970s from the writings of Dr. Broda Barnes, who felt that patients with both low body temperatures combined with many symptoms of thyroid deficiency clearly benefited from thyroid treatment. Unfortunately, Dr. Barnes's work fell mostly on deaf ears. By the late 1980s, however, Dr. Denis Wilson picked up that thread and refined it with the use of a specially compounded, long-acting thyroid medication. This form of thyroid deficiency evaluation and treatment now often carries his name.

Here is the idea of Wilson's syndrome: under certain conditions, the thyroid gland produces enough hormones so that all blood measurements are normal. However, on a cellular level, the body may not be able to utilize this hormone properly. Thus, the body actually behaves as if it is thyroid deficient, even though the blood tests might come back normal. We have learned a number of mechanisms by which this may happen, making it an increasingly more scientific concept. What this means is that if a patient comes to my office with fatigue, constipation, weight gain, brain fog, and low body temperatures, even if her blood tests are normal, she may well need to take thyroid hormone to heal. So if no blood test can accurately diagnose Wilson's syndrome, then how can we diagnose it? Well, there's only one way to clarify things: a trial of thyroid hormone administration. If patients respond clinically with clear improvement, they have it; if not, they don't. It's pretty much that simple.

Unfortunately, in my experience, it is the rare physician who is willing to provide thyroid hormone on a trial basis. I don't know why. This is not a dangerous treatment, and having provided this on a trial basis to 3,000 to 4,000 patients, I am convinced of its safety and efficacy. In all this time, we have had only rare and minor side effects, with no reactions of significance.

Part of the difficulty in finding a physician willing to try this is that conventional practitioners, especially endocrinologists, have already dismissed this concept as bogus, without actually trying it. I am aware that every single endocrinologist in southwest Missouri would dismiss this concept out of hand, as being unscientific and unfounded. I am not aware that a single one of them has tried this on a single patient, which would make that dismissal just as unscientific. I readily admit that before I tried this form of treatment, I was also skeptical. But the immediate and profound number of success stories was overwhelming, to the point that it became clear: this is a very valid, very useful concept and treatment.

I am certain that thousands of patients with treatable thyroid problems are undiagnosed every year by our profession and go untreated. And because patients are untreated, they continue to suffer, needlessly. Let's look deeper into why this is the case by examining just how the thyroid works.

Thyroid Function

The thyroid gland makes two hormones, triiodothyronine and tetraiodothyronine, nicknamed T3 and T4. The 3 and 4 refer to the number of iodine atoms in the molecules. T3 is considered the active hormone, meaning it's the one that does all the work for us. Thus, T4 must be converted into T3 in order to be effective. This is where the problem starts.

Under a variety of stressors, the body may lose its ability to convert T4 into T3. This means that patients have seemingly sufficient amounts of thyroid hormone available, but that they unfortunately cannot convert those hormones, on a cellular level, from T4 into the T3 they need. Thus, to all intents and purposes, these patients behave physiologically as if they are lacking T3 on a cellular level, and truly are deficient in the thyroid hormone they require. Another important consideration is that both thyroid and estrogen hormones are transported through the body by the same carrier protein. This means that imbalances in estrogen hormones can, and do, affect the amount of thyroid hormone available to the body. The kinds of stressors that can create this imbalance, which Dr. Wilson refers to as "resetting the thyroid thermostat," include both physical stressors such as major surgery, severe infections, and childbirth, as well as emotionally intense stressors. Remember, from the body's perspective, stress is stress. Once the thyroid mechanism has been disturbed, it may stay that way until it's treated.

Treatment

Since the problem with thyroid deficiency is T3 production, the usual thyroidal treatment of T4, referred to as *Synthroid* or *Levothyroxin*, could be seen from this discussion as neither logical nor optimally effective. The treatment should obviously be administered as T3. Now, there is a medication that has been available for years called Cytomel, which is a synthetic form of the T3 hormone, but it doesn't last very long in the body when provided in its usual form. To make things even more complicated, patients are extremely diverse when it comes to how quickly their bodies can metabolize Cytomel. Some patients need to take it every four hours to keep a decent level in their system, while others can take it every eight to twelve hours, with every imaginable variation in between. Dr. Wilson recognized this difficulty during his research, so he got a compounding pharmacy to create a long-acting T3 product that would slowly and steadily release the T3 into the body over a twelve-hour period. We abbreviate this as LA T3 (Long Acting T3), and it must be produced by a pharmacy that is knowledgeable and capable of compounding it (not your usual pharmacy). These *compounding pharmacies* are staffed by pharmacists who have received additional training in order to be able to prepare these compounded products, and they require additional facilities in order to prepare these properly. Some patients already on T4 who do not feel their bodies are in balance may need to switch to T3, using this method until they get back into balance.

The important thing to remember is that even when your blood tests are completely normal in regard to thyroid functionality, you could still experience low body temperature, fatigue, constipation, weakness, and changes in hair texture. If this is the case, you might be a suitable candidate for a trial treatment of LA T3. But how can you tell if you have a low body temperature, short of just measuring it a few times? Well, you might have to do a little bit of math. I recommend to my patients that they take their temperature four times per day by mouth (using an oral thermometer), for at least a week, and then calculate the average of those numbers. Unless the temperature average is 97.8 degrees or less, it is unlikely that we're dealing with Wilson's syndrome. It is more accurate if the patient can find (and read) an old-fashioned glass thermometer.

In my office, when patients come in and are already on the T4 treatment, I wean them off for a week and then begin a new protocol. For those who have never taken thyroid medication, or those we are switching from T4, I start by having them take tiny doses of LA T3 twice a day, and then slowly increase the dose every three days. During this time, we carefully monitor both physical symptoms and temperature. When we reach the correct dose, patients usually respond immediately. If a patient truly has Wilson's syndrome, there will be an obvious, often dramatic, improvement when we reach the optimal dosage that balances his chemistry. This will be demonstrated as a significant improvement in symptoms and a corresponding rise in body temperature. Usually my patients can put an actual value on their response to treatment, and I've had them report anywhere from a 20 to 80 percent improvement in overall feeling and health. Since patients are so biochemically different, the dose required (and hence the number of dosage increases attempted by the patient) will vary considerably. Please understand that this discussion is an over-simplification of a more complicated treatment, and should not be attempted without professional and expert guidance.

Now here's the best part: once patients have responded, they can usually take that dosage for three to six months, be weaned from it, and then never need thyroid treatment again. If they are already on thyroid treatment, they often will need a lower dosage and will feel much better following this treatment. Unless the thyroid gland has already been permanently damaged, this is not a lifetime treatment, as it would be for those with damaged glands. This particular treatment is a rebalancing program, and once completed, the body usually remains in balance. On rare occasions I have seen patients relapse after an intense stress brings the deficiency back. However, I would estimate that 60 percent of the patients I try this with respond beautifully, which makes this a much more common deficiency than most physicians suspect.

As I reiterate throughout this book, the proof of this concept lies not in theory, but in patient response. The only way doctors can make this diagnosis is to *try* the treatment. How a human being responds to treatment is the truth for that particular patient. Be aware, also, that there are other approaches for treating the thyroid gland, most notably Armour Thyroid, which is a combination of T3 and T4. However, in my experience, the LA T3 is much more effective in this regard.

Tanya's Story

Thirty-nine-year-old Tanya came to my office in June 2008 with complaints of fatigue, a constant headache, a generalized achy feeling all over her body, and some degree of depression. She had experienced fatigue even as a teenager, but as a teacher and a mother, she couldn't live that way. She told me that if she could, if she were allowed to, she would lie in bed all day. Starting with her early history of fatigue, she got significantly worse after the birth of her first child. She was given Prozac at that time, which helped a little, and she was told at various times that her thyroid was just sluggish. Modest amounts of Synthroid were of minimal benefit to her. After the birth of her second child, six years before she came to me, Tanya went downhill again. She had recently undergone a hysterectomy and she made it perfectly clear to me that she was having problems: "I am a raging bitch."

I began by measuring Tanya's DHEA level, and it was quite low at only 161 ng/dL (normal for her age is about 750 ng/dL). I started her on 50 mg of DHEA each morning, and put her back on a small dosage of Prozac. By her second visit, six weeks later, she was only a little better. Because her problems were clearly not stemming from just her DHEA deficiency, I asked Tanya to get an average measurement of her body temperature. It averaged 97.7 degrees, almost a full degree under the normal temperature. Along with her other symptoms, this low average temperature made Tanya an excellent candidate to try a course of LA T3 as a treatment for what I presumed to be Wilson's syndrome. At the second visit, after realizing that DHEA was not her only deficiency, I put her on the LA T3 protocol. When she reached a dose of 45 mcg of that compound every twelve hours, she noted immediate improvement, and five weeks later she reported that she was "better in every way."

Tanya now gets up each morning motivated and energetic, and she was able to move her entire classroom at the start of the school year without getting exhausted. "I can really tell a difference," she told me. She rated her improvement from the time we started the treatment at 80 percent. The enhancement in her overall attitude and demeanor was dramatic. "I'm actually happy now," she said. "And I'm not glued to the couch all day anymore." Her headaches are virtually gone.

We are looking at the relief of years of fatigue, depression, and headaches, after only five weeks on this method of thyroid treatment.

❖

While most of these patients' stories are rather complicated, here is a nice example of how quickly this simple intervention sometimes works wonders.

Ellie's Story

Ellie, forty-six years old, was referred to us through some of her co-workers, who were also patients of ours. Her primary concerns were that of fatigue, and she rated her energy level as three on a scale of zero to ten. She also reported a severe abdominal pain that had begun just recently. We were able to address the abdominal pain with methods that will be addressed over the next two chapters, but the fatigue was a different animal altogether.

I noted that she had normal thyroid blood tests, but that her temperatures averaged 97.6 degrees. So I offered her a trial of LA T3, and she discovered that by taking a tiny dose of medication, 7.5 mcg of this hormone every twelve hours, she sustained remarkable improvement. Within a few months, Ellie's energy level had improved to the point that she was ready to discontinue her thyroid medication completely. She reported that she was really pleased with her progress and felt that her energy had come back to normal.

Here is an excellent example of how a simple trial of a tiny dose of thyroid medication, even in the face of normal thyroid blood tests, produced impressive results that could not have been achieved unless we had given it a chance.

Iodine Deficiency: The New Frontier

For those of us who live in the Midwest, it has long been known that iodine deficiency is rampant. The soil in this region is so severely depleted in iodine that crops grown on this soil and the animals that feed on those crops are all iodine deficient. Nearly 100 years ago, medical professionals realized that the common presence of an enlarged thyroid gland in the form of a goiter was due primarily to this deficiency of iodine. To counter it, iodine was added to salt, creating iodized salt.

The incidence of goiters diminished greatly, and we reached a place where everyone just knew that iodized salt had to be a part of our daily lives.

This practice continued for decades, until the 1980s, when cardiologists began to emphasize the possible problems of consuming too much salt, most notably because of its effects on high blood pressure and heart disease. At about the same time, bread manufacturers removed iodine from their product and replaced it with bromide. Over time, what we created for ourselves was a double whammy. That is, we now have a serious situation where iodine intake has once again dropped dramatically, especially in the Midwest. An informal poll of my patients, most of whom are holistically oriented, shows that over 90 percent of them mostly consume sea salt. While perhaps a healthier form of salt intake, sea salt also does not contain iodine. The other part of this double whammy is that our environment now contains large amounts of fluoride and bromide. Both of these elements are so similar in structure to iodine that they bind to the sites in the body that require iodine, and essentially block it from functioning. So we have evolved a situation in which we have inadequate amounts of iodine in our diet, and the small amount that we do take in cannot function properly because of the presence of fluoride and bromide.

Until recently, we have not had the ability to accurately test for iodine levels in our bodies. But over the past several years, a few labs have developed the Iodine Load Test, which enables us to learn with a great deal of accuracy whether patients are deficient in this key element, and to what extent. The test is relatively simple to perform: patients take an oral measured dose of iodine with potassium iodide, and then collect all of their urine for twenty-four hours. If they have a sufficient amount of iodine already, then the dose we give them will pass right through their system and into their urine. If they are deficient, their bodies will grab the iodine they need, and that iodine will not make it into the urine. A normal test would show that 90 percent or more of the iodine administered made it into the patient's urine. Anything less than 90 percent denotes varying degrees of deficiency.

In my own practice, I have found that over 90 percent of my patients are significantly iodine deficient. Replacing the iodine is simple and often produces great clinical improvement.

Iodine is taken up by the body mostly through the thyroid gland, so any thyroid imbalance should also address the patient's iodine needs. That is why I am including this discussion in this chapter. The other major tissue of the body that needs iodine is the breast. It is less commonly appreciated that breast problems may require iodine replacement as well. This is true for fibrocystic breast disease and for the prevention and treatment of breast cancer as well.

Recent research suggests that iodine is needed in every cell of the body for its optimal metabolism. As our knowledge about iodine deficiency expands, I suspect we will be looking at a global problem, not unlike the one that existed 100 years ago. We will need to re-learn to add iodine back into our diet.

Estelle's Story

Estelle was forty-seven years old when she came to me because of her struggles with fibromyalgia and chronic fatigue. She had many of the problems which accompany fibromyalgia, including irritable bowel syndrome, depression, and menopausal symptoms. She had symptoms that suggested that mold toxicity might be part of this constellation as well. Throughout this book we will discuss the various methods of diagnosis and treatment of these conditions.

Estelle's health did improve noticeably with our complete treatment approach utilized in our office. However, she was still not well enough to return to work and was still barely functioning and somewhat depressed. When I performed the Iodine Load Test, I discovered that her levels of excretion were only 59 percent (normal being 90 percent or more). Within six weeks of starting the use of iodine and potassium iodide (Iodoral), Estelle was markedly better. Her depression had lifted, and her energy level had improved to such an extent that she was able to resume full-time work.

I hope that you're beginning to see how this whole functional medicine model works: we analyze, step-by-step, the likeliest imbalances in the body, treat them, and see how the patient responds. With each response, we add another piece to our understanding of the puzzle. If the patient does not respond to our intervention, we stop it and go back to the drawing board to come up with the next viable puzzle piece. The vast majority of our patients are far too complicated for one single treatment to cure them. Instead, what you will see is that we keep building on our successful treatments until the patient has crested some threshold, unique to themselves, and becomes well.

Further Reading

Arem, Ridha. *The Thyroid Solution: A Revolutionary Mind-Body Program for Regaining Your Emotional and Physical Health.* New York: Ballantine, 2007.

Brownstein, David. *Iodine: Why You Need It, Why You Can't Live Without It.* 2nd ed. West Bloomfield, MI: Medical Alternatives, 2006.

Wilson, E. Dennis. *Wilson's Thyroid Syndrome: A Reversible Thyroid Problem.* 4th ed. Rice, WA: Cornerstone, 1991.

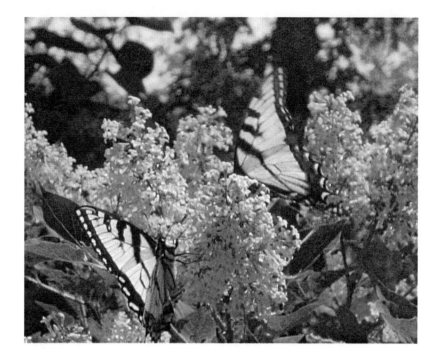

Chapter 6

Sex Hormones

Now That I Have Your Attention . . .

I'm afraid this chapter won't be as racy as the title suggests. In fact, the sex hormones are quite similar to some of the other hormones we've already talked about, like the thyroid and adrenal. It's simple: you need them, and you need them in exactly the right amounts. This is not one of those cases where more is better. Thyroid balance is perhaps a more obvious example, because we know that taking too much of that hormone is not good, but having too little isn't good for us either. Other hormone levels follow this same rule. Like Goldilocks's porridge, they have to be *just right*. Sex hormones follow this same model.

Estrogen Deficiency

Certain tissues in our bodies are designed to interact with hormones preferentially. That is, these tissues have specially constructed landing sites called *receptors*, each of which is designed to respond to specific hormones and not much else. For example, in women there are receptors for the estrogen hormones located in the brain, heart, and vaginal tissues. These receptive tissues *need* estrogen in order to function properly. Without it, the brain simply doesn't work as it should, and when estrogen levels are low, we see the symptoms of estrogen deficiency that are listed below:

- Hot flashes
- Night sweats
- Mood swings
- Depression
- Insomnia
- Fatigue
- Cognitive impairment (difficulties with focus, memory, and concentration)
- Vaginal dryness
- Urinary frequency and urgency
- Decreased libido (sex drive)

Several times a year I will see a woman who has seen her cardiologist for heart palpitations but with no solutions to that problem. Often, when we provide estrogen for a measured deficiency in that hormone, the palpitations disappear. Vaginal dryness is frequently the result of the body lacking enough estrogen to meet the needs of those tissues. While hot flashes and night sweats get a lot of press and attention, they are not as important for a woman's health as these other considerations. To put it a bit differently, while hot flashes are really annoying at times, and while many women do suffer through them quite terribly, a woman's inability to think clearly or sleep well or her sudden, inexplicable outbursts at her family are, medically speaking, far more serious. Just think of it: a woman who is irritable when she knows she has no reason to be, who cries over small things, who is depressed and can't sleep, who cannot think clearly or truly function in her daily life, has a serious but readily treatable problem. In terms of health, again, these items are not luxuries, but necessities, as any woman who is going through this will tell you.

We have, of course, been aware of menopausal difficulties for centuries. In ancient China, menopausal women would drink the urine of pregnant women to treat these symptoms (pregnancy results in a dramatic increase in estrogen production). However, in our current medical climate, somehow, these hormones have become charged with a great deal of misinformation. Many women (and men) are reluctant to take hormones because some physicians have suggested that they will be at a higher risk for a host of serious diseases. The most current concern is that estrogen will cause cancer, especially of the breast, and bring patients closer to heart attacks, strokes, and gall bladder disease. Let's be clear about what is being discussed.

Several years ago it was finally accepted that Premarin, the most widely prescribed medication in the United States, was clearly associated with a significant increase in breast cancer and blood clots. I say finally because we had plenty of information about this link for many years prior. In fact, four years have passed since this alarming fact first came to light, and we've noted that the incidence of breast cancer has dropped by almost 20 percent! Premarin, short for PREgnant MARes' urINe, is actually a synthetic material, a third of which consists of several types of naturally occurring human estrogens, while the other two-thirds consist of mostly horse estrogens called equilins. So for years doctors had been giving huge numbers of women synthetic materials, most of which were foreign to their metabolism. They coupled that prescription by adding synthetic progesterone, also foreign to their metabolism. Why should we be surprised that this turned out to be an unhealthy combination of synthetic hormones, a concoction we recommended to women for years?

News of the dangerous side effects of synthetic hormones finally came to light, and it scared millions of women. The medical profession made a complete reversal of position. For years previously, the profession had implied that all women who were going through or had completed menopause needed to take these synthetic materials. Doctors believed that not only would these materials make menopause easier for women to tolerate, but that they would also protect against heart disease and perhaps Alzheimer's disease. As we know now, they do nothing of the sort. Hormones are an integral part of a very fragile, delicate balance in the body. So why would an unnatural, synthetic chemical be of such great benefit? When the medical profession suddenly stopped prescribing these materials, women got scared. Many, without even consulting their physicians, stopped their synthetic hormones cold. Medical professionals scrambled for an answer for those millions of women who were now struggling with the frightening symptoms listed above. The best immediate answer for many women, according to conventional medicine, was to take a particular type of antidepressant: specific serotonin reuptake inhibitors (SSRIs). This was the pharmaceutical industry's answer for millions of women suffering from estrogen deficiency. While those medications can, indeed, help somewhat with the symptoms of depression, mood swings, sleep, and hot flashes and night sweats, they are purely symptomatic treatments; what a woman's body needs is estrogen, and these medications are but a weak substitute for the real thing. Conventional medicine has not entirely abandoned Premarin, but rather reserves it for use only in the most severely afflicted women, knowing now its risks.

There is another answer to this problem, and it is one that conventional medicine has been slow to embrace, again for reasons I cannot fathom. We have available, and have had for years, *natural hormones*: estrogens, progesterone, and testosterone, which are concocted and made available through compounding pharmacies. These materials are now commonly referred to as *bioidentical* hormones, meaning that they are biochemically identical to the hormones we make for ourselves. Bioidentical hormones are generally extracted from plants, which, surprisingly, produce the same hormones we do. These bioidentical hormones have not been studied as long and carefully as the synthetics; in fact, I don't anticipate that they will be, since research dollars come primarily from the pharmaceutical industry, and you cannot patent— thus make huge profits from—natural materials. The research we do have, however, indicates that the bioidentical materials are much safer and better tolerated than the synthetics. From my perspective, that makes a great deal of sense, as natural materials would obviously suit the body's needs most effectively than would synthetics.

I personally view hormone replacement as a physical need that must be met. All symptoms are just the body's way of telling its owner that something is not right and something must be done. How could that be wrong? I've provided natural hormone replacement for over fifteen years, and my experience is that it is very safe, very well tolerated, and very necessary. Why would you take an antidepressant when your body really needs estrogen? I cannot count the number of women I've treated who are living comfortable, productive, and healthy lives using natural hormones. This includes those who had done poorly on synthetic hormones, as well as those who have chosen to go directly to the bioidentical materials.

One unique aspect in the prescription of natural hormones—which has never been characteristic of conventional approaches to synthetic hormones—is that I start by measuring the current hormone levels with a simple blood test. Most physicians have found that blood testing of these hormones is much more accurate that salivary testing. That, too, is my experience. This blood test gives me a precise idea of what the patient needs. I can then write a prescription for exactly that amount of hormone, and this prescription will be filled by a compounding pharmacy. This precision is really helpful. For many years, Premarin came in only two dosage strengths: 0.6 mg and 1.25 mg. This never made sense to me. Given the biochemical uniqueness of all women and of all people in general, how could only two choices of dosage meet all of their individual needs? Years later, Premarin was made available in two additional dosages of 0.3 mg and 0.9 mg. Even so, only four dosage strengths for all women?

After we measure the levels of the three estrogens, estriol (E3), estradiol (E2), and estrone (E1), as well as progesterone and testosterone, we can design a natural hormone replacement that precisely puts that woman back into balance. Philosophically, it makes sense to me that meeting a woman's personal, unique hormonal needs is a healthy thing to do, and my experience reveals that this is true. Women who were unable to take Premarin for a variety of reasons, including migraine headaches, joint pain, and a host of more subtle side effects, can usually take the natural materials with no side effects at all.

We still have much to learn. How to formulate these bioidentical hormones is an area of debate among physicians. I've noticed that capsules work best for most of my patients. Some physicians prescribe the hormones as capsules designed to be placed into the cheek and left until they dissolve, which are called *troches*. Other physicians administer the hormones using topical creams, but many of us have found that absorption of hormone from the skin is quite variable, and I've found that topical creams are not as reliable or predictable as capsules. Nevertheless, natural hormones are much safer than synthetics and much more appreciated by a patient who needs them to function, no matter the form in which they are taken.

As with any hormonal treatment protocol, the patient needs to be followed carefully by someone trained in using these materials. Patients should never begin any natural hormonal treatment without the supervision of a knowledgeable clinician or medical practitioner. In this digital age, it is possible to go online and have bioidentical hormones shipped to you without putting a healthcare provider in the loop. I've had patients come to me already taking these materials, and they are usually struggling because they had no idea about dosage or balance. Again, this makes little sense to me. You wouldn't take thyroid hormones or insulin without an expert's guidance—why should this be any different?

Progesterone and Testosterone for Women

Having focused on estrogen thus far, let's expand our discussion into the other hormones, first with women, and then with men.

All hormonal health is about *balance*. Somehow, the public has gotten the idea that it's all related to estrogen levels. When a woman is in her prime, hormonal health concerns every one of her hormones, so why would that change when she gets older? The time in which a body is moving into menopause but hasn't quite gotten there is called *perimenopause*. We have learned that this stage involves an imbalance called *estrogen dominance*. In evolved menopause, we see clear estrogen deficiency, but before the ovaries stop making much estrogen, there is a time in which it makes even less progesterone. When this occurs, symptoms arise because there is way too much estrogen *relative* to progesterone. The estrogen is dominant, the balance is tipped, and this is quite unhealthy. Many women who experience this assume that they just aren't making enough estrogen, but actually the reverse is true. When we evaluate this balance by hormone testing, we can provide natural progesterone until the hormonal shifts into true estrogen deficiency. We can also measure testosterone, which is needed primarily for energy and sex drive. With our measurements, we can custom-make a prescription at any phase in this process that will enable our patient to be in balance, and we believe that this translates into health.

Many women fear that they will have to take hormones forever. This is rarely the case. Most find that after several years they have outgrown the need for hormones and will not need them again. Part of the process of treatment is for the patient to periodically stop taking hormones to see how she responds. Her body will tell her, quite clearly, whether or not she still needs the bioidentical prescription.

It is also helpful for patients to be aware of the important interaction of estrogen with thyroid hormones; not only that, but estrogen's interaction with all of these hormones and the adrenal hormones, along with serotonin and dopamine. This means, as I'm hoping to convey, that we shouldn't look at one hormone in isolation, but only in relationship to other hormones. We must maintain balance. These are biochemical dominoes. One deficiency begins, affects another, and then another, and then another. These hormones are an important and integral part of our Big Six approach to the evaluation of biochemical imbalances in the body.

Kristy's Story

Kristy was forty-three years old when she came to see me several years ago, and she had a very simple request: "Fix me." She told me that she had been on low doses of thyroid hormone for twenty-two years, but she still felt like she had all the symptoms of thyroid deficiency. The most prominent of these was extreme fatigue. She described lying around in bed all day without much movement. On a bad day, she would get up and try to do laundry, pay bills, and clean her house. But this would end up exhausting her. "My body throbs and muscles pain all the time," she told me.

When Kristy awoke in the mornings, it was as if she had been beaten with a baseball bat all night. It often took her until noon for her to be able to get up and get dressed. She did not have hot flashes or night sweats, but she did have significant problems with focus, memory, and concentration. She also had vaginal dryness and an unusually low sex drive. She admitted that she was irritable and angry all of the time and felt depressed. The problem was that she knew she had nothing to be depressed about.

Kristy had undergone a hysterectomy eleven years earlier, but her ovaries had been left intact. It is quite frequent after any gynecological surgery for an early menopause to ensue, but most physicians believe that it's nearly impossible for a woman to begin her menopause until she is in her late forties. Unfortunately, these complaints of early menopause often go unrecognized and unheeded.

The standard test used by conventional medicine to determine the presence of menopause is called the follicle-stimulat-

ing hormone test (FSH), but many physicians are unaware that this test may not turn out positive results until five to eight years after menopause has actually begun! This huge chunk of time completely misses the diagnosis, and the opportunity to help that unfortunate patient is lost in the confusion.

For Kristy, laboratory testing showed low progesterone, estriol, and DHEA levels. I supplemented her with 25 mg of DHEA each morning, and I also put her on a compounded prescription of estriol and progesterone to increase those levels. Her thyroid testing came back entirely normal. This was interesting, as she had been taking thyroid hormone for so long.

When she came back for her six-week follow-up visit, Kristy told me that she was doing really well, about 85 percent better than before. She had gone off the thyroid supplements without any negative effects, so it was clear that her rapid improvement was due to the use of hormones and DHEA. She only got sore, or tired, after really overdoing it, and essentially felt she was close to being cured in just six weeks.

Testosterone in Men

While it receives much less attention, there is also a male menopause. Men also have estrogen and progesterone in their bodies, but in far smaller concentrations than women. For a variety of reasons, one of them being the excess aromatase enzyme made in fat cells, men may convert some of their testosterone into estrogen. When this happens, their hormone balance is altered. Too much estrogen can affect male sexual functioning, and just as important, energy and stamina. A little-known but vital fact is that a great deal of research shows a man's testosterone level profoundly affecting his heart. The higher the testosterone level, the less likely a man is to have a heart attack. This, too, has received little attention from conventional medicine.

We continue to be deluged with advertisements for Viagra, Cialis, and Levitra. These medicines have, indeed, enabled many men to function sexually at a much higher level, and they are quite useful in that respect. But they don't help the body to make more testosterone, which is probably what it really needs.

So, as with women, we need to be measuring testosterone levels in men, as well as estrogen levels and other binding proteins that allow us to determine what the true balance point is. Then, we can provide natural hormonal replacement when indicated. Unfortunately, many athletes have abused the use of testosterone and its precursors, so the FDA has made testosterone a *scheduled* drug, placing it in the same class for prescription as narcotics. In no way does that change the biochemical need that a man may require to achieve normal hormone levels. The following list illustrates the most common symptoms of testosterone deficiency:

- Fatigue, tiredness
- Decreased stamina
- Decreased libido (sex drive)
- Erectile dysfunction
- Muscle weakness
- Depression
- Mood swings
- Hot flashes
- Palpitations
- Insomnia
- Inability to concentrate
- Antisocial tendencies

In this culture, it is perfectly acceptable for women to discuss their hormone balance with their doctors. Unfortunately, there is a form of stigma or reluctance for men to do the same. I suspect that many men could live much healthier lives if they could just understand that these are natural biochemical alterations, and that there is as little shame in noting sexual changes as there would be in noting the onset of diabetes. Both need treatment. Alas, many men suffer not only sexual dysfunction, which they will not discuss with anyone, be it their doctor or best friend, but they also experience the consequences of decreased energy levels, stamina, and muscle weakness, which are just as serious.

Sheldon's Story

Sheldon came to see me when he was forty-two. Initially, his symptoms consisted of extreme fatigue and an overall sense of feeling poorly. We quickly realized that he had developed adult onset diabetes mellitus, and with conventional treatment, he rapidly improved. But after several months, he was still aware of residual fatigue, poor stamina, and a decreased sex drive with moderate erectile dysfunction. When we tested his testosterone level, it was quite low at 178 ng/dL (normal level is 241-827 ng/dL). I have often found that in younger men, the indiscriminate use of testosterone may, because of its biofeedback loops with the pituitary gland, actually shut down the production of testosterone and paradoxically make the problem worse. Instead, I provided Sheldon with a prescription for a small dose of Clomid, 10 mg, taken three times weekly, which stimulates the testes to make more testosterone. Follow-up measurements of his testosterone levels showed that they had come back into the middle of the normal range, and he reported immediate improvement in energy, stamina, and sexual function. (His wife, also a patient of ours, thanked me too).

As I hope you see, for both men *and* women in poor health, investigating this aspect of hormonal balance is another central feature of our program.

Further Reading

Morgenthaler, John, and Jonathan V. Wright. *Natural Hormone Replacement for Women Over 45*. Petaluma, CA: Smart, 1997.

Shippen, Eugene. *The Testosterone Syndrome: The Critical Factor for Energy, Health, and Sexuality—Reversing the Male Menopause*. New York: M. Evans, 2001.

Vliet, Elizabeth. *Screaming to be Heard: Hormonal Connections Women Suspect, and Doctors Still Ignore*. 2nd ed. New York: M. Evans, 2000.

Chapter 7

Food Allergies

Nothing to Sneeze at . . .

You might think it's somewhat obvious: the food we eat, the water we drink, and the air we breathe play an especially significant role in our overall health. Unfortunately, the basic concepts of nutrition and digestion, as well as their importance to health, are not only given little attention in medical school education, but they are often neglected or ignored in current clinical practice, as well. When patients ask their doctors about these subjects, they are often given the impression that these things don't matter much. But they do matter—a lot. The patient's discomfort, in fact, is directly connected with the discomfort of the healthcare provider. These patients realize that their doctors don't always have the information that they are seeking. But why not? Aren't they medical specialists?

Over the next few chapters, I would like to discuss several medical concepts that are not parts of conventional medicine. These include food allergy, the overgrowth of toxic microorganisms (bacteria, yeast and parasites) in the intestinal tract, and then how food may stimulate the over-production of insulin in the form of hypoglycemia (low blood sugar). But first, we turn to food allergy.

Immediate Sensitivity vs. Delayed Sensitivity

There are several different kinds of food allergy. Each is unique because of the various antibodies produced by the body in response to its reaction to a particular food. All of our allergies crop up based on how our immune system reacts to a specific material, usually a protein. There are five specific and different kinds of antibodies that the body can create, and they are all called *immunoglobulins*. They are differentiated by letters, so we call them Immunoglobulin A (IgA), as well as IgD, IgE, IgG and IgM.

Perhaps the most common type of food reaction with which most of us are familiar occurs when someone consumes a particular product (commonly seafood, strawberries, or peanuts) and then breaks out into hives within fifteen to twenty minutes. This alarming reaction by the immune system is brought about by the specific immunoglobulin IgE. All physicians acknowledge the importance and existence of this reaction. If severe, in fact, this reaction can result in life threatening conditions in which the lips and tongue swell up and the ability to breathe becomes compromised. We call these types of responses *immediate sensitivity reactions*. They constitute medical emergencies and must be treated as such.

More common in patients, but much less known within our profession, are the *delayed sensitivity reactions*, which are mediated primarily by immunoglobulins IgM and IgG. These reactions can produce a wide array of symptoms and illness with the delay ranging from six hours to three days. This delay makes these reactions much harder to diagnose because most of us don't remember what we ate three days ago and are not likely to attribute what we're feeling today to something that we consumed that long ago. These reactions, however, are quite prevalent, and they are indicated in the following list:

- Fatigue
- Arthritis or arthraligia
- Bronchospasms
- Allergic rhinitis
- Eczema
- Cholecystitis
- Heart palpitations
- Enuresis (bed wetting)

- Cognitive difficulties
- Myalgia
- Inflammatory bowel disease
- Irritable bowel syndrome (IBS)
- Psoriasis
- Urinary frequency and pain
- Autoimmune disease
- Sinusitis

Clarence's Story

Clarence was a seventy-four-year-old gentleman who came to me several years ago complaining of a sudden increase in joint pain, which was diagnosed by his family physician as arthritis. Along with his joint pain, which he experienced all over his body, he also noted an increase in fatigue and poor concentration. I asked Clarence if he was eating more of any particular foods than usual. He responded that since it was summer and fresh corn and tomatoes were now available in abundance from his garden, he was eating those foods almost every night. As these are common allergic foods, I suggested that he stop eating tomatoes and corn for ten days. It usually takes three days for the intestinal tract to clear what is already in it from recent meals, so I cautioned him that he might not see any results for that time. I indicated to him that if these foods were indeed the cause of his symptoms, he should experience rapid improvement by eliminating their intake. To his surprise, at his next visit he informed me that his symptoms had resolved completely.

I then instructed Clarence to test these foods separately by eating a lot of the one food we suspect as our allergic culprit with every meal for three days. If he did not react, he could try the next food. If he did react, he should wait for three days to clean the system out and try the next one. He discovered that he reacted to both of them. Tomatoes and corn brought his symptoms back with full force, but those symptoms disappeared again when he stopped eating those foods. Not only did his joint pain vanish, but he felt much more energy,

and his concentration came back to normal as well. This is an
excellent example of classical delayed food allergy.

Diagnosis and Treatment

I would estimate that at least 50 percent of all joint and muscle pain is caused by food allergy, and when the offending foods are discovered and their consumption discontinued, many patients feel much, much better. This means that a great deal of what is commonly diagnosed as osteoarthritis or degenerative arthritis is actually a food allergy reaction. It also means that it is readily treated by discovering the offending foods and avoiding them. The diagnosis of *arthritis* is far overused by physicians, which is quite unfortunate. It is defined to patients as an inflammation of the joint, with the implication that it is permanently and ultimately destructive to that joint. Arthritis is a frightening word that creates pictures of life-long suffering in patients' minds. As I am implying here, however, this is actually not often the case, since joint allergy pain goes away readily and completely when the offending substance is removed from the diet. A more precise medical term for this form of joint pain would be *arthralgia,* which simply means "joint pain," and does not carry the implications of destructive, eternal, or long-lasting pain. Occasionally, medical practitioners unwittingly cause additional suffering to their patients by an imprecise use of language, and this is a good example of how that can happen.

The commonest foods incriminated in the delayed food allergy reactions are cow's milk and wheat, followed in terms of frequency of reactions by sugar, corn in all of its various forms, and citrus products. Additional foods that can often specifically affect joint pain are pork and the nightshade family of plants, which includes tomatoes, potatoes, egg plant, and green peppers. Although Clarence's story involved the symptom of joint pain for these delayed allergies, please keep in mind that any, or even several, of the symptoms present in the above list could react and respond in this way, both to evaluation and treatment.

Once delayed food allergy is suspected or considered as a possible component of any illness, there are several ways to make a clear and accurate diagnosis. The simplest and cheapest, though not necessarily the easiest, method is to embark on what we call an *elimination diet*, which I explained in Clarence's story. This type of diet consists of eliminating all of the most likely offending foods and observing what happens over time. Typically we continue this elimination process for seven to ten days. As I noted above, the first three days of this diet are unlikely to give us much information, since the intestines have not yet expelled all of what is already in the system. So we really focus on the four to seven days after the elimination diet has begun. All I ask my patients to do is observe how they feel on this diet. If their symptoms improve or resolve significantly, this means that one or more of the foods we've eliminated is causing those symptoms, and we have established food allergy as a probable diagnosis for their illness. From here on, we have to play Sherlock Holmes to figure out which food or foods are the culprits.

Usually we eliminate all of the likeliest offenders at once. This means that I ask patients to stop consuming all milk products, wheat and corn in all forms, sugar, citrus, and any other food they suspect may be contributing to their symptoms. When I present this plan to my patients, some express that they would rather do this one food at a time, so as to make the process a bit easier for them. But I discourage this. The reason for encouraging patients to discontinue all of the likeliest foods at the same time is that many patients have *multiple* food allergies. For example, if a patient is allergic to both milk and wheat, and she eliminated the wheat but continued to consume milk, she could miss the benefits of being off wheat because the milk was still producing an overriding allergic reaction. Although it is a bit more troublesome for the patient to eliminate all possible offending foods simultaneously, it is a much more accurate method for evaluating response.

If after seven to ten days, with a careful and meticulous elimination diet, the patient notes no improvement whatsoever, it is unlikely that those foods are a part of the problem, and I then encourage the patient to resume his usual diet. This does not completely rule out food allergy as a part of the problem, but it does tell us about those specific foods we just tested.

On the other hand, if the patient is clearly better (not necessarily cured, as there may be other components to the symptoms), then we must understand which foods are responsible. The simple rule I work with is for the patient to add back one new food, lots of it, in pure form, every three days. Let's go over this in more detail. To ensure the highest level of accuracy, we test with only one food in pure form. This means that if you are testing milk products, you can consume lots of milk, cream, yogurt, sour cream, or cottage cheese. This does not include foods such as ice cream, which contains sugar and flavorings. Eating non-pure foods would compromise the interpretation of the patient's response. Delayed food reactions, as I have noted, may take up to three days to show up, so we have to wait at least that long to be sure that no reaction has occurred. If a reaction occurs sooner, of course, the patient should discontinue that food immediately and wait three days to clear it out of her system before testing another food.

Delayed sensitivity reactions also require that enough of the tested food be eaten to produce a reaction, if there is going to be one. Tiny amounts may not produce a noticeable reaction. Along with the three-day delay, this is another reason that intelligent, thoughtful patients have not suspected food allergy as a component of their symptoms. For example, if patients ate Wheaties for breakfast, a sandwich for lunch, and pizza for dinner, they might not recognize that they are consuming a substantial amount of wheat. Smaller amounts of wheat, say just the sandwich for lunch, might not produce this reaction, which would throw otherwise observant patients off track. They might notice that sometimes they reacted to wheat and sometimes not. Quantity matters, especially when doing this type of testing.

Sometimes, less commonly consumed foods, even in trace amounts, are the culprits, and these can be difficult to diagnose. In the past, tests for food allergy such as skin testing and radioallergosorbent (RAST) blood tests have been used, but they are quite inaccurate. In recent years, ELISA technology has improved the situation considerably. The most accurate test I've found is the ELISA/ACT blood test performed by Dr. Russ Jaffe's laboratory. He uses a somewhat unique testing procedure on blood, evaluating for exposure to 380 common foods and 100 common household chemicals. By using the results produced by his laboratory, I've enabled many of my patients to improve or heal. Additionally, materials that are more difficult to test for, such as food coloring and additives, can be discovered with this test. The chemical monosodium glutamate (MSG), frequently used as a meat tenderizer or flavor enhancer in Chinese restaurants and steak houses, is a common allergen. Increasingly, we find that Nutrasweet (aspartame) also causes delayed sensitivity reactions, especially in migraine sufferers. Dr. Jaffe published a paper on the prevalence of food allergy in fibromyalgia, noting that 73 percent of those patients had significant food allergies, and that their symptoms responded well to the elimination of the offending foods.

Olivia's Story

Olivia was seventy-six when she came to me with a long, twenty-five-year history of the inflammatory bowel disorder, Crohn's disease. This condition can be a serious, life-threatening medical problem. She had been followed by gastroenterologists at the University of Kansas medical school, and she received all of the customary biopsies, clearly confirming the diagnosis, and underwent the customary treatments. Nevertheless, she had never done well with these conventional treatments. Upon testing her stool, I found pathogenic bacteria and yeast (infective microbes), which we treated (see the next chapter). I also identified her food allergies and we removed those offending materials from her diet. Olivia's symptoms resolved completely for the first time in twenty-five years. She was absolutely thrilled. When she returned to her gastroenterologist for follow-up colonoscopy, he found no trace of her bowel disease.

When Olivia described our treatment program to her gastroenterologist, who had followed her for years, he told her it was impossible that this treatment could have led to her remission. I guess it was possible that our treatment wasn't a factor in her healing. However, since she has continued to do extremely well, with no recurrence over the past eight years, I can be reasonably comfortable in concluding that her exceptional improvement occurred because we removed the allergic foods from her diet that were directly responsible for bringing on these symptoms. She still finds that if she mistakenly eats one of the foods she reacts to, she will have a short episode of symptoms, but no full-blown recurrence of inflammatory bowel disease has re-appeared.

❖

Norma's Story

Norma first came to see me at the age of forty-two with the diagnosis of rheumatoid arthritis. She had been seeing a rheumatologist and three other physicians for the past several years, but over the past year had not responded to any of the eight or nine medications prescribed. She hurt all the time and she was frustrated. Norma was one of those unfortunate patients I see occasionally who had severe reflux problems from a sensitive stomach, and almost all the medications that had been used to treat her rheumatoid arthritis had flared up those gastrointestinal symptoms intensely. She had gamely tried every medication available for treatment, but each one had severe, intolerable side effects. She was hoping that a completely different approach might be of value.

To digress for a moment from the subject of food allergy, we have found with rheumatoid arthritis, as with several other autoimmune conditions, that a number of alternatives are often helpful. As we describe here, looking for and treating food allergies is often an effective strategy. Additionally, looking for and treating heavy metal toxicity is often of value, and the use of long-term, low dose minocin (an antibiotic in the tetracycline family) has been effective for some. Newer information about the benefits for the immune system by treating vitamin D deficiency has also emerged. And, as unusual as it sounds, there is a long history for the use of bee venom in treating this condition. There is even a report in the medical literature that describes the use of journaling, in which patients spend twenty minutes a day, for just three days, writing down on paper a detailed account of their stressors and their feelings about those stressors. This simple procedure for many patients results in significant improvement, and fortunately for Norma, she responded well to this method (see Chapter 21 on autoimmunity).

Another area of benefit to Norma came from our culturing her stool, which we will discuss at length in our next chapter. I discovered the presence of the pathogenic bacteria Klebsiella on her stool culture, and we treated it. Klebsiella is especially associated with joint pain, so looking for and addressing it is often helpful for patients with that affliction.

After completing and treating Norma's pathogen problem, we then utilized Dr. Jaffe's ELISA/ACT test, which showed that she had strong delayed reactions to aluminum, chocolate, cocoa, black tea, cinnamon, coconut, polysorbate 80 (a common food additive), tapioca, chili, orange, caraway seeds, saccharine, paprika, shrimp, cola, sage, basil, and several household chemicals. Let me point out here that not only can aluminum be a toxin, but here it was an allergen as well.

When she meticulously avoided all of the foods and chemicals denoted by her testing, Norma reported astounding improvement in her symptoms. For several years afterward, her rheumatoid arthritis was well controlled with careful monitoring of her diet and occasional treatments of osteopathic manipulation. When she would get a flare-up of symptoms, she often recognized that it was because of particular stressors. By utilizing the journaling technique for several days to let out these particular stressors, she would often feel much better.

As Dr. Jaffe has discovered, and I can confirm, many autoimmune diseases have a food allergy component. Patients with rheumatoid arthritis, lupus, and multiple sclerosis have improved significantly—and some have even been cured—by uncovering this component of their illness. In my experience, food allergy is one of the most commonly overlooked causes for a wide variety of symptoms. Countless children with eczema and asthma and enuresis (bed wetting), and adults with joint pain and fatigue, headaches, colitis, and irritable bowel syndrome have greatly improved with this simple evaluation. We will also look at the role food allergy plays in autism spectrum disorder later in this book.

With this discussion and these few examples, you can immediately begin to see how important food allergy's role is in causing or contributing to any chronic medical condition. Many patients are astonished to learn that some of the foods that they regularly eat are actually a part of their problem, and that the simple expedient of avoiding these foods provides great benefit. We regularly observe, to our patients' frustration, that the most likely allergic foods are the ones that they identify as their favorites. Of all the ideas presented in this book, food allergy is one of the commonest and often easiest to address. It's truly a shame that its importance is not universally recognized.

Further Reading

Breneman, James C. *Basics of Food Allergy*. 2nd ed. Springfield, IL: Thomas, 1984.

Crook, William G. *Tracking Down Hidden Food Allergies*. 2nd ed. Jackson, TN: McGraw-Hill Professional, 1980.

Chapter 8
Intestinal Dysbiosis

Alimentary, My Dear Watson

The next really useful concept that is not yet a part of conventional medicine is that of *intestinal dysbiosis*. The word dysbiosis comes from "dys," reflecting an imbalance, and "biosis," pointing to the life forms or microbes which normally inhabit our intestines. Hence, this difficult but accurate phrase conveys the sense that the flora and fauna of our gut are out of balance. Essentially, I am referring to the complicated ecosystem of our gastrointestinal system, which we will cover in more detail here. Understanding the workings of this complex system provides doctors a method for evaluating this particular part of our physiology so that we can improve or heal it. Let me flesh out this concept a bit more.

The Gastrointestinal Tract

Although we don't usually think of it this way, our gut is really a giant open tube, connected to the outside world through the front end (our mouth) and the back end (our rectum). The gastrointestinal tract is seemingly inside of us, as seen from one perspective, but from another perspective, it is also outside of us. It cannot possibly be sterile or free from germs like the rest of our body, because it is constantly in direct contact with the external environment. When we eat food or drink liquids, those materials mix with the secretions of this giant tube, allowing our body to digest and assimilate what it needs. Because our gut is not sterile, meaning that it is filled with bacteria and other germs, we have evolved a very complicated ecosystem that actually helps us in many ways as we interact with both good and bad bacteria, yeast, and other microorganisms that gain entry into this system.

Our body actually *needs* a significant quantity of bacteria to populate the gastrointestinal tract for a variety of reasons. For one, since this is a true ecosystem, the more numerous the beneficial bacteria are, the less of a foothold is available for the more toxic (*pathogenic*) bacteria to gain space or nutrients in which to grow. Another reason we need these good bacteria is because they manufacture a number of nutrients that we need to survive, such as vitamin B-12. Rather than be upset or concerned about the presence of these bacteria, we should instead know that they are an integral part of our healthy bodies, meaning we coexist with them in a way that is beneficial to both of us: we need them, and they need us. If this system is disturbed or damaged, most commonly by our taking antibiotics that kill off large numbers of helpful bacteria, the ecosystem is imbalanced. Destroying these beneficial bacteria allows room for the pathogenic bacteria, yeasts, and parasites, to gain a toe-hold and grow. Depending on which species of pathogen infects us, we may experience a variety of gastrointestinal symptoms: heartburn, reflux, gas, bloating, distention, cramps, pain, diarrhea, or constipation. Additionally, many of these pathogens release toxins into our body, which can cause us to feel systemically, or globally, ill. Fatigue, depression, joint pain, cognitive impairment, and headache are just of few of the symptoms which may be due to the out-of-balance growth of bacteria or yeast within our intestines.

Furthermore, approximately 60 percent of our immune system is found connected to our gastrointestinal system. This portion of the immune system is called the *gut-associated lymphoid tissue* (GALT). Surrounding our gut are large patches of lymphocytes (important immune cell lines) called *Peyer's Patches*, which process any potentially harmful microbes. The Peyer's Patches produce antibodies to invaders and immunoglobulin A to create a major line of defense. When you think about it, it isn't surprising that our body places so much emphasis on an immune system so close to our gut. Remember, we are dealing with an open-ended tube to the outside world, a system that is constantly exposed to possibly infectious agents. It makes sense that our bodies would have evolved this elaborate arrangement for dealing with these potential dangers. Our body has surrounded its intestinal system with a good portion of its immune system, assigning to that system the specific mission of monitoring the gastrointestinal tract and defending it from the invasion of potentially harmful germs.

If the invading microorganisms produce toxins or create an infectious or inflammatory response in the intestinal cells, it can weaken the tight connections between the intestinal cells, which are an important form of protective barrier. Once these cell-to-cell connections have been loosened or opened by inflammation, the toxins can enter our body to do damage. This is also the mechanism by which food allergy occurs: we can only develop a food allergy if a foreign protein makes its way into our body without our blessing. The only way for these proteins to get across the barrier is to seep through the weakened cellular connections, which are supposed to be tight junctions. Other parts of our immune system are then forced to make antibodies to these proteins, hence causing food allergy. This disturbance in the tight junctions is often called *leaky gut*.

The Second Brain

Another important and often under-looked component of our gut physiology is called by some scientists our *second brain*. For many years, we have known that there is a larger concentration of neurotransmitters in the gut than there is in the brain. Neurotransmitters are chemicals that allow electrical impulses to be conducted from nerve cell to nerve cell, and we will discuss them at length in our chapter on amino acids. Neurotransmitters include some chemicals of which you may have heard: serotonin, dopamine, and epinephrine. Recent research points to our intestinal tract as contributing to our mental well being by its production of these neurotransmitters, yet we still don't know exactly how this works. Old phrases such as "gut feeling" and "gut instinct" take on completely new meanings in this context.

This interaction in our intestinal system of good bacteria, the GALT, and neurotransmitters creates a complicated, interwoven system that we are just beginning to understand. The phrase *intestinal dysbiosis* is intended to convey some sense of that complexity, and provides us with a great tool to analyze and understand it. Ultimately, this can help us to heal, especially if this area has been neglected or damaged.

The Intestinal Tract as an Ecosystem

When I describe the gastrointestinal tract as an ecosystem, many of my patients look puzzled and confused. So allow me to use a bit of poetic license and paint a picture of what this ecosystem might look like. Imagine that your intestinal tract, both the small and large intestines, consists of miles and miles of white sandy beaches, with the ocean lapping up gently along its length. Populating these glorious beaches are thousands and thousands of happy families, the children diligently building sandcastles while their parents wade into the surf or lay out on brightly colored beach towels. Imagine also the fringes of these beaches, way back in the dunes or hidden in small groves of trees behind the beach, where we might discover a few wild animals lying in wait—coyotes, raccoons, even a bear or two. These animals are extremely suspicious of the many humans roaming around, and they choose to remain in hiding. But when the sun finally sinks below the horizon, when the beaches are less populated, these beasts come out in search of food. In this picture, the people represent the good bacteria, consisting of many species of *Lactobacilli* and *Bifidobacteria*, the main species of good bacteria that populate our small intestine and large intestine, respectively. The wild animals represent different kinds of toxic species, such as *Candida* and pathogenic, or toxic, bacteria. This would be our healthy, normal state.

Now, imagine that something occurs to interfere with that perfect day at the beach, say, a shark attacking a man while he surfs. Our happy families will leave the beach in droves, fearful that the shark might get another bite out of someone else. This mass exodus of people gives those wild animals complete and comfortable access to our beach. The indiscriminate use of antibiotics can be quite a shark attack for our body's beaches because they kill off so many good bacteria. What antibiotics leave behind are those wild animals, those creatures with no place else to go. In turn, the animals will eventually begin to grow and thrive. Our beaches will become populated by coyotes and raccoons and bears, and the families with their children will be very reluctant to come down to the beach ever again. The animals, those toxic species, have gained the upper hand.

When we attempt to rectify this situation, we use specific medications and herbs that could be seen as clearing the beach of all sharks. These treatments invite thousands of new families (a symbol for the use of probiotics) to come down to the beach and play. The wild animals have been happy at this beach for some time now, but they are now being driven off, slowly but surely. They migrate further and further down the beach until the families feel safe enough to return. That this is a slow and gradual process of change during treatment is important to understand: we can't simply get into beach jalopies and ride wildly onto the sands, shooting indiscriminately at the wildlife. Instead, we have to work *with* the system to restore it. As you might imagine, this does take a little time. I hope this little analogy, although a bit fanciful, will help you to understand the concept of intestinal ecology.

Diagnosis

In practice, when we encounter situations like this, I first ask my patient to collect a stool specimen (a bit disgusting, but truly helpful), and I send it to a laboratory for analysis. Over the years, I've had excellent results from the Genova Diagnostics (formerly called the Great Smokies Diagnostic Lab), but many others can provide these analyses as well. From the information derived from the stool specimen, I can determine whether or not the patient's body can make enough digestive enzymes and hydrochloric acid, or whether some form of malabsorption of certain food nutrients is taking place. Most importantly, from this analysis I can determine if there are normal amounts of good bacteria in the intestines, including *Lactobacilli*, the main beneficial bacteria of the small intestine (which many people associate with Acidophilus), and *Bifidobacteria*, the main beneficial bacteria of the large intestines. From these test results, I can also evaluate for the presence of toxic or pathogenic bacteria, yeasts, and parasites. In a healthy patient there should be plenty (designated as 4+ on the lab report) of both the *Lactobacilli* and *Bifidobacteria*. If the patient has received significant exposure to antibiotics, even in the distant past, the antibiotic may have upset the delicate balance by killing off the good bacteria and leaving small amounts of toxic microbes behind to multiply. The overgrowth of this toxic bacteria or yeast can persist for years.

The toxic bacteria irritate, infect, or inflame the intestines, causing or contributing to irritable bowel disease, spastic colon, and inflammatory bowel diseases such as Crohn's disease and ulcerative colitis. Additionally, these microbes can release toxins into the patient's body that can contribute to chronic fatigue, brain fog, joint pain, and headaches. All of these symptoms are usually accompanied by an overriding sense of not feeling well, which goes well beyond simply bowel symptomatology. The good news is that the laboratory not only tells us which microbes are involved, but it also tests these microbes against the known antibiotics and natural remedies that could destroy them. This is similar to the well-known process that doctors use when patients report that they have a bladder infection. A sample of their urine is tested for what are called "culture and sensitivities." That just means that doctors take the urine sample, place it on a culture plate, and set discs of the most useful antibiotics on top of the sample. The discs that clearly kill the growing bacteria obviously represent the antibiotics we want to use to treat that infection. In exactly the same manner, we can use culture techniques to determine the best treatments available for the specific microbe we find on our patient's stool test.

One of the things we've learned over the past several years is that these organisms that infect our bowel are mutating and becoming less and less sensitive to the medications we have used against them for a long time. In conventional medicine, the concept of chronic yeast infection is not considered to be a valid diagnosis when it refers to a species of *Candida* found in our intestinal tract (it can also occur in the vaginal area). As with other concepts discussed in this book—hypoglycemia, dental amalgam toxicity, chronic Lyme disease, chronic Epstein-Barr infection, and food allergy—the medical profession has somehow decided to ignore the presence of yeast in the gastrointestinal tract. Some do so by claiming that everyone has small amounts of yeast, so it's nothing we need to pay attention to. Some have disparaged this concept by confusing it with *systemic yeast infection*. Systemic infections are caused by those yeasts that have gotten into the blood stream and are delivering toxic microbes to every part of our body. Systemic yeast infections certainly exist, but they are very rare, and, when present, are life-threatening. A patient with this type of infection requires intravenous antibiotics and hospitalization. But this is not what we are discussing here; instead, we are discussing overgrowth of yeast and toxic bacteria specifically in the bowel. While these overgrowths are not life-threatening, the direct inflammatory effects of these micro-organisms coupled with the release of toxins, which make their way through the bowel wall into the rest of our circulation, can make us feel pretty wretched. If these are not diagnosed and treated properly, we can feel this way for a very long time. Those physicians who maintain that these overgrowths are of no importance are missing an opportunity to make a big difference in their patients' intestinal health.

Many patients associate the word "yeast" with vaginal yeast infections. While these infections are quite common, they are not exactly the same as intestinal yeast infections. Both cause patients to feel poorly; in one, the intestinal symptoms predominate, and in the other, vaginal symptoms predominate. The difference is that the "leaky gut" associated with dysbiosis allows toxins to be absorbed into the body and adds another level of toxicity for our patients. This does not happen with vaginal yeast infections

Once again, by observing how patients respond to treatment, we can learn of the importance of this condition. Healing is not about theory; it's about results. I have personally treated several thousand patients who had an overgrowth of yeast from the intestinal system, and all of these cases were confirmed with the stool analysis. Nearly all of these patients report significant improvements in their symptoms from treatments. If intestinal yeast is such a normal state of affairs, as many conventional doctors tend to believe, how could this healing be possible? When we repeat the stool tests of successfully treated patients, the *Candida* is no longer found. Might it still be present in miniscule amounts? Yes, it could be, and probably is. After years of looking at these results, I am strongly persuaded that any overgrowth noted on this test represents a non-physiological state, and patients who demonstrate these laboratory results will benefit from our treatment.

Treatment

The results of our recent testing, as I alluded to above, show that the yeasts are getting less responsive now to our older treatments. As the media has been actively informing us about how many species of bacteria are evolving ways of no longer responding to our usual antibiotics, yeasts are doing the same thing. Years ago, a variety of simple medications such as Nystatin, and herbs such as capryllic acid, garlic, and berberine were quite effective at killing intestinal yeast. But as we continue to observe the results of these sensitivity tests, we find that herbs now rarely control these infections. Nystatin, in particular, is increasingly less effective than it used to be, and we have to turn to stronger anti-fungal medications for results. Even Diflucan, our old standby, no longer works in 10 to 15 percent of patients. Other stronger medications like Sporanox and Ketoconazole have become a necessity for successful treatment.

The key point I wish to make here is that by doing a simple stool test, which is covered by most insurance companies, we can identify and treat these infections with precision. We simply follow the sensitivities provided by the laboratory and then add back the nutrients and supplements that we identify to be deficient. Usually treatment involves adding probiotics, enzymes, or hydrochloric acid, accompanied by a change in the patient's diet.

Probiotics

Probiotics are various combinations of good bacteria, like the *Lactobacilli* and *Bifidobacteria* mentioned above. Many probiotics include additional ingredients to improve the body's ability to nurture these good bacteria. These ingredients include fructooligosaccharides (FOS) and the benign yeast *Saccharomyces*. Here is where a trained, knowledgeable health professional comes in. Some of the pathogenic bacteria we are trying to defeat thrive on FOS, and the incorrect or indiscriminate use of probiotics and their additional ingredients without testing can lead to serious problems. This should not come as a surprise. Doctors can treat the condition properly if they know more precisely which bacteria and yeast are involved. It keeps coming down to this: a clear and concise diagnosis is necessary for an appropriate treatment. Otherwise, we are just shooting in the dark, and we might get lucky, or we might not. Why shoot in the dark when light is available?

There are a bewildering number of formulations of probiotics and an equal number of opinions on how to make the best use of them. Many beneficial bacterial species present in probiotics are killed, or mostly killed, by stomach acid. This means that a large proportion of these bacteria, if ingested in tablet or powder form, do not reach their intended destination alive. It also means that when my patients tell me that they are getting plenty of good bacteria in the commercial yogurt and acidophilus milk they consume, they may be mistaken. When we look at their stool tests, many are surprised to discover how few good bacteria are actually present in these products. Logic and experience, therefore, suggests that the best way to deliver these beneficial bacteria to our intestines would be through an *enteric-coated capsule.* This protection would ensure that the capsule goes through the stomach acid unscathed and dissolves in the intestines, placing the beneficial bacteria exactly where they need to be.

Another common form of delivery of these bacteria is through freeze-dried bacteria. These bacteria are processed so that they are not really alive until they are reconstituted in the intestines. While many of the makers of these products claim superb reconstitution, our stool tests do not bear this out.

The best results seem to come from *live culture* bacteria, which, by definition, require refrigeration. These are not as convenient as the freeze dried form, which can sit out at room temperature for long periods of time, but in my opinion the freeze dried variety are nowhere near as effective as the live bacteria.

Rochelle's Story

Rochelle came to me in 2004, complaining of weight loss over three months, accompanied by severe abdominal pain. She reported that three months prior, she had developed the onset of a dull pain in the left side of her abdomen. She had been told three years previously that she had diverticulosis, and she had her gall bladder removed. After that, she seemed to be much better. However, three weeks before she came to see me, while eating breakfast, she all of a sudden felt very faint. She felt bloated and didn't even want to finish her meal. She rested up for a few days and began to feel a little better.

Several mornings later, again while eating breakfast, Rochelle noticed a pressure in her upper stomach. She became very shaky inside and felt dreadful. Her blood pressure had increased to 190/90, so she went to her local emergency room for evaluation. There she was given an antibiotic for a presumed recurrence of her diverticulitis, despite the fact that her pain and discomfort were caused by a burning sensation in her upper-to-mid stomach area. (Diverticulitis typically involves pain and symptoms in the left lower quadrant of the abdomen.) Blood tests and x-rays were taken but did not clarify the diagnosis.

Rochelle settled down for a few days but then had another episode very similar to the previous ones, with the new onset of loose, watery diarrhea. She was given Lomotil, and although it did improve her diarrhea, it also set off an increase in abdominal cramping. Rochelle had lost fifteen pounds in only two weeks, and she found that Zantac helped a bit to decrease her stomach pain. When we treated her with Nexium, a somewhat stronger antacid preparation than Zantac, she noted no benefit and continued to experience severe symptoms and lose more weight.

I performed a comprehensive stool analysis and found that Rochelle's body was not digesting fat properly. It also wasn't making enough stomach acid, had low stores of butyrate (a necessary nutrient for colon cells), and most importantly showed an overgrowth of two different species of Candida. With this information, I started her on betaine hydrochloride to replenish her hydrochloric acid. I also had her take calcium butyrate and digestive enzymes rich in lipase with each meal. I added Diflucan to kill the yeast and placed her on a high-protein, low-carbohydrate diet so that she would not keep feeding the yeast. Carbohydrates are nutrients that feed the yeast, so depriving the yeast of its sustenance is essential to its elimination.

Rochelle responded well to this regimen, and within a month she was markedly improved, with only occasional stomach aches and diarrhea. With the resolution of the abdominal pain, we reviewed the concepts of an elimination diet to look for food allergy as a component of her symptoms. We also began the medication Librax, a bowel calming product. Within a few more weeks Rochelle was completely well. She has continued to do well in the five years since, and as long as she watches her diet and takes her supplements, she is a happy camper.

Rochelle's story is an excellent example of how severe irritable bowel syndrome can be successfully treated by using these concepts. The majority of patients with this disorder can experience dramatic improvement by looking for intestinal dysbiosis and food allergy and treating it. There is often a stress component to irritable bowel disease, and it helps if we address this as well.

When patients come to my office with unexplained intestinal symptoms and have already had a full evaluation, which usually includes a CT scan of the abdomen and upper and lower endoscopy, most of them can benefit from investigating dysbiosis and allergy. You might want to review Olivia's Story from our last chapter to better understand the uses of this treatment process.

Nathan's Story

Nathan's mother and father brought this nearly two-year-old child to my clinic almost ten years ago. Nathan wasn't gaining weight normally and had become very irritable and fussy in his first year of life. Just before I saw him, he had been admitted to a university-based pediatric hospital for three full weeks, diagnosed with pneumonia and what we call "failure to thrive," which simply means that he wasn't growing at a normal rate. Despite intensive evaluation in the hospital and the use of hyperalimentation (a process in which intravenous proteins and lipids are used to help supplement the nutritional process), Nathan had still lost another pound. His parents described Nathan waking up at night with what seemed to be stomach pain and gas, noting that one night he had awakened and screamed for three hours. As they reflected on his symptoms, his parents were beginning to think that eating cheese may have played a role in his symptoms. (He had been breast fed for eighteen months and clearly got worse after beginning to consume milk products.)

Nathan also had sporadic bouts of diarrhea and frequent episodes of asthma and eczema (a skin rash often associated with allergy). When we checked his stool test, he had a severe overgrowth of Candida and almost no Lactobacillus present. So we treated the yeast overgrowth with antifungal agents, provided a good supply of probiotics, and took him off all milk products. He begin to improve immediately, and slowly over several years he moved up the growth chart from below the fifth percentile (meaning really poor growth) to the twenty-fifth percentile, which represents significant improvement. The eczema disappeared, and his asthma improved as well. I have had the opportunity to watch Nathan grow into a fine youngster, and his bright eyes and demeanor are a far cry from the sunken skin and dull eyes of his first visit.

In our next chapter we will discuss blood sugar and its role in health. Hypoglycemia is really about another area of intestinal physiology and fits in nicely with this discussion, so it seems to me that the flow of information should place it next in our awareness. As this will begin our next section, which I call the "Little Six," you might wonder why certain discussions merit a "Big" designation, while others are "Little." Please understand that these names are meant to simplify the process of looking at the complex interweaving of these ideas. The "Big Six" is just my designation for the six most commonly overlooked components of chronic illness, and the "Little Six" is my pet name for the six next most common components. It doesn't mean that any of these are less important than the other (particularly for individuals in which one piece of information may prove pivotal in their cure); it just means that I typically start with the first six, as they are statistically the most likely to be a useful starting point for a given patient. We then move into the next grouping if that evaluation does not provide the healing we seek.

So onward and . . . onward.

The "Little Six"

opefully, you've now discovered a great deal about the most common imbalances that may be contributing to your illness. With a little luck, identifying and treating these factors might have cured or greatly improved your health. I sincerely hope that you are now so far along the path of healing that you don't need to dig any deeper.

Unfortunately, many of my patients, while considerably better and thrilled with their improvement, still need me to dig deeper into their imbalances and find more to treat.

I call the second phase of this process The "Little Six." These are the next most common deficiencies and imbalances that we will pursue. The order in which I do this, as before, depends on the details of my patient's history, and we will go after the most likely culprit first.

This section starts with the commonly under-diagnosed condition of low blood sugar, also referred to as hypoglycemia; that will be our Step 1. Then we will turn to the area of dental toxicities, which includes mercury toxicity, imbalances in the electrical charges on different teeth, and root canals, Step 2. The newly recognized realm of mold toxicity and its larger arena of biotoxicity will be covered in Step 3. This will be followed by the related area of unrecognized chronic infections (which often contribute to biotoxicity) and includes viral and bacterial (especially Lyme disease) species in our Step 4. Amino acid deficiencies, particularly because of their importance in building up our neurotransmitters (so important for treating depression and anxiety) will be Step 5. Our newest addition, which has added another dimension to our treatments, is that of evaluating and treating methylation defects, in Step 6.

The vast majority of my patients are much better, often cured, when we have completed these steps. But not everyone gets better. The labels of the "Big Six" and the "Little Six" might imply that once we have completed this process of evaluation, we have looked at everything that can possibly go wrong; alas, this is not so. In his book, *From Fatigued to Fantastic!*, Dr. Teitelbaum's identifies over 150 imbalances known to contribute, at times, to the cause(s) of fibromyalgia and chronic fatigue. The good news is that no one has all of these imbalances. However, this information does underscore the fact that there can be a lot more than twelve steps to healing.

It is my hope that I can, in these pages, provide legitimate hope for healing, by explaining, and at times oversimplifying a complicated process. Medical detectives must be willing to be patient, thoughtful, and diligent in sifting through the clues we have collected to provide a precise diagnosis for our patients. It is through correct diagnosis that we can move toward healing. So please be aware, from the beginning of this journey, that we may need to keep on digging to find your pay dirt.

When we have completed all of these steps, whether you are better or not, know that there is still much more we can do for you. I have not tried to cover everything we have learned, since I fear that this would overwhelm you, but be aware that there is a great deal of hope for you in the information we have acquired.

Let us take off now on the next leg of our journey ... the "Little Six."

Chapter 9

Hypoglycemia: The Myth and the Reality

Sugar in the Morning, Sugar in the Evening . . .

*I*n the mid 1980s, patients who were inexplicably ill began to read about a mythical creature called *hypoglycemia*. The warnings about this creature were dire: an encounter with it would bring about fatigue, brain fog, difficulty with focus and concentration, shakiness, heart palpitations and sweating, and an overall feeling of discontent. This beast would completely conquer your body, and its presence was explained by the presence of low blood sugar, thus giving it the moniker, *hypoglycemia* (*hypo* means "low," and *glycemia* refers to sugar in the blood). The science and reality of low blood sugar has been well described since we were first able to measure blood sugar years and years ago. We know that if diabetics take too much insulin or oral medication, their blood sugar can drop to dangerously low levels, so low that they could pass out while walking or driving. We also know that some newborns are particularly prone to low blood sugars and must be treated aggressively as having a serious medical condition. In fact, at one point in time, hypoglycemia was defined in medical practice as a blood sugar level of 50 mg/dL or lower. This was accepted as standard medical knowledge for decades.

However, a sizeable group of patients began to realize that their symptoms seemed to correlate with their low blood sugars, and they began to visit primary care physicians by the droves. An odd phenomenon occurred: physicians were uncomfortable with the vague nature of these complaints and what they perceived to be an overall difficulty in managing these patients. There was a clear overlap of these symptoms with anxiety. Heart palpitations and tremor, which are frequent components of hypoglycemia, are often reported as symptoms of anxiety. Many primary care physicians were uncomfortable treating anxiety, preferring to refer those patients to psychiatrists. In a rather perverse attempt to alleviate physician discomfort, at a great disservice to patients everywhere, several papers were published by endocrinologists in which hypoglycemia was renamed *reactive hypoglycemia*. The implication of this new name was that low blood sugars were really a sort of laboratory glitch that didn't represent a true biochemical event. Hence, the presence of a measured low level of blood sugar could be dismissed out of hand as unimportant or irrelevant. This was wonderful news for many physicians who could then inform their patients that they only had reactive hypoglycemia, which had no medical significance and needed no treatment. Unfortunately, it also dismissed, out of hand, the presence of very real (not imaginary) low blood sugars that were significantly affecting the health of many patients. This placed them in the position of being told that they should seek psychotherapy for what was actually a physical problem.

Patients were informed, therefore, that these symptoms were to be ignored, and were to be labeled as *psychosomatic*. Now this is an interesting word. All it really means is that the mind (*psyche*) and the body (*soma*) are one. If something occurs in the body, say, low blood sugar, it affects the mind by directly causing fatigue and difficulty in mental functioning. This is a clear description of what happens to us physiologically, not psychologically. Unfortunately, the meaning of psychosomatic has shifted to something it was never intended to convey: that the symptoms are not real and exist only in the mind. That is how the diagnosis of hypoglycemia became a myth. With only a little twist of language, the field of medicine summarily dismissed thousands of patients who were struggling with the symptoms of hypoglycemia, and they simultaneously removed any hope of improvement. This is nothing to be proud of, and, regrettably, this misunderstanding persists to this day.

The following list illustrates the most significant symptoms of hypoglycemia:

- Fatigue
- Weakness
- "Brain Fog" (inability to think clearly)
- Tachycardia (rapid pulse rate)
- Diaphoresis (sweating)
- Shakiness and tremor
- Anxiety
- Syncope (passing out, when hypoglycemia is severe)

My understanding of low blood sugar is fairly simple: if patients have some, or all, of the symptoms of hypoglycemia, and also have a low blood sugar level drawn at the time they are experiencing these difficulties, then low blood sugar is probably the cause of their symptoms. Even clearer, if we treat it and the symptoms resolve, then as far as I'm concerned, they have this diagnosis and we're correctly treating it. It really is that simple, at least for me and for my patients. No efforts to explain it away or dismiss it out of hand make any sense to me.

The symptoms experienced by each patient depend largely on the actual blood sugar level, and patients vary in their sensitivity to these levels. Some patients are exquisitely sensitive to minor drops in glucose, and others can tolerate it somewhat better. There is actually a spectrum of symptoms, based on blood sugar levels. So with small drops in blood sugar, the patient is likely to experience fatigue, brain fog, and difficulty with focus or concentration. As the blood sugar drops further, this may proceed to sweating, heart palpitations and tachycardia (rapid heart rate), and as the blood sugar levels drop even further, to tremors and full blown anxiety. I suspect that a large number of patients diagnosed with panic attacks and anxiety actually have undiagnosed hypoglycemia.

What is really at fault here is that the patients with this problem have what I call a "trigger-happy pancreas." What lowers our blood sugar as it starts to rise when we eat a meal is the secretion of insulin by the pancreas. For patients with hypoglycemia, their pancreas produces too much insulin, and it drops the blood sugar well below the normal levels. (I will graph this out for you later in this chapter.) Unfortunately, we cannot promise a cure for hypoglycemia, as the tendency to have a hyper-reactive pancreas producing too much insulin is usually life-long. The good news, however, is that we can treat or manage it quite well. In the best of cases, we can prevent the most serious complication of hypoglycemia: diabetes. It would seem logical that if hypoglycemia is produced by an excessive release of insulin from the pancreas, over time this would eventually exhaust or deplete the pancreas's ability to make insulin, resulting in diabetes. This can and does happen in a significant percentage of patients with hypoglycemia. But if we *prevent* the pancreas from being over-taxed, with proper treatment, the chance of this developing into diabetes can be reduced drastically.

When patients arrive in my office complaining of fatigue or exhaustion, especially in relationship to when they eat their meals, I start to pay close attention. They rarely recognize the problem until we bring it to their attention because they usually assume it is coming from something external. I begin asking them about the potential relationship between the timing of their meals and the onset of their symptoms. Do they get sleepy or tired or weak two hours after lunch? If these symptoms persist and these patients begin to feel shaky or sweaty or they experience heart palpitations, do they feel better after they eat? Many patients have learned to consume sugar regularly (especially soft drinks and candy) throughout the day in order to avoid these symptoms of low blood sugar. But they are unwittingly making themselves worse.

Karl's Story

When I first met him, Karl was a 35-year-old engineer who complained of extreme fatigue to the point of depression. In fact, he thought he was depressed and noted that for the previous ten years, he had been unable to motivate himself to build his business. This was somewhat surprising to him since he'd been a "go getter" all his life and thought of himself as a high-powered individual. As he began describing his difficulties to me, Karl admitted that he really didn't recognize himself anymore. It was like he was just going through the motions of life in a kind of fog.

I started by conducting some basic lab work on Karl, including DHEA and magnesium tests, both of which returned normal results. I then gave him a five-hour glucose tolerance test. This test measures a patient's blood sugar level every hour for five hours after consuming a measured amount of glucose. (We will go over this test in more detail soon). It documented that he had a profoundly low blood sugar, which occurred three hours after consuming the glucose load of the test (which is similar to how the body reacts after eating a meal). So I put him on a program which consisted of a high-protein, low-carbohydrate diet and included the consumption of high-protein, low carbohydrate snacks at two-and-a-half hours after each meal, to help prevent the drop in blood sugar that we now knew would occur at three hours after eating a meal. Just three days later, a completely different Karl stepped into my office. He was bright-eyed and bushytailed, no longer morose and down, and he told me that his vitality had completely returned. He was no longer depressed, and he was taking on every project in sight with new enthusiasm.

I have followed Karl for the past ten years, and as long as he eats properly, he is highly motivated and successful at his work. Every once in a while, when he gets sloppy about his diet, symptoms recur, and that is a clear message for him to get back to the diet that he knows works so well for him.

Over the years, I have treated hundreds and hundreds of patients like Karl. Most, like Karl, are stunned to discover that if they eat correctly, they can feel amazingly better. Years of malaise can simply melt away.

So here's how it works. When I suspect that a patient might be suffering from hypoglycemia, I perform a standard (but rarely done) five-hour glucose tolerance test. A single blood sugar level, taken at only one time of the day, is not adequate to tell us what we need to know. Keep in mind that blood sugars normally fluctuate throughout the day, and at any one moment in time, that lab test merely reflects the levels at *that* precise moment. Patients respond in unique ways to processing glucose, and a low blood sugar can appear anywhere from one to five hours after we begin the test. Some practitioners even use a six-hour test, but I have not found that extra hour helpful, and it unnecessarily prolongs the testing.

The patient visits her local laboratory after eating nothing past midnight the evening before. Consuming water is fine, but no food or coffee should be ingested from midnight until the time the test begins. The lab begins by drawing a blood glucose level while the patient is fasting, which is used as our baseline level. The patient is then given a drink containing 75 gm of glucose. After consuming this drink, the lab simply measures the patient's blood glucose every hour for five hours. From the patient's perspective, this is an annoying and sometimes difficult test, because if she truly has hypoglycemia, she might get weak, shaky, and anxious during the test. However, if the patient does experience those symptoms at the same time that we find a low blood sugar, it becomes a very useful test, as it often provides information we couldn't otherwise obtain. It is not unusual for patients to discover, when we graph the results of their testing, that a great number of their symptoms are finally explained. I will often hear: "Wow, now I understand why I feel so lousy two hours after lunch." Perhaps more important, when patients see their altered physiology in a black-and-white laboratory report, they begin to realize that their symptoms are not psychological.

When we perform this test, the baseline glucose level is typically 90 mg/dL, and a normal person will usually respond to this glucose challenge with a rise in his blood sugar levels to up to 160 mg/dL at one hour, which then drops back down to 90 mg/dL at two hours. Figure 9.1 shows how we look at it over time. The vertical axis represents the level of blood glucose, and the horizontal axis demonstrates time, starting from baseline at "0" and moving up through the five hours of the test.

What's really happening here, as we described previously, is that in response to a rise in blood glucose, the pancreas senses that rise in glucose and must respond by producing exactly the right amount of insulin to bring that blood glucose back to baseline.

Now let's look at what a hypoglycemic patient's graph might look like. Figure 9.2 shows that even with the same baseline, a patient with hypoglycemia has what I have referred to as a "trigger-happy" pancreas. The pancreas of a hypoglycemic patient, in response to the rising blood sugar level (produced by the carbohydrate provided by a meal) produces too much insulin, too soon. This excessive amount of insulin doesn't allow the blood sugar to rise as it normally would. Even more important, the insulin produced in excess by the pancreas plunges the

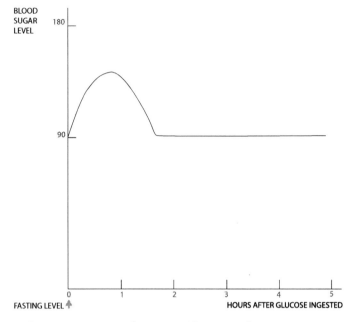

FIGURE 9.1   Normal 5-Hour Glucose Tolerance Test

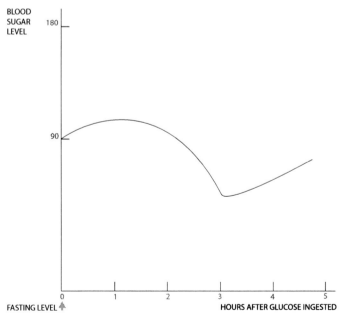

FIGURE 9.2   5-Hour Glucose Tolerance Test in Hypoglycemia

blood glucose level, which stays down until it can pull itself together and get back to baseline.

Although the medical definition of hypoglycemia is that of 50 mg/dL, I have found that even blood glucose levels in the 70s can represent true hypoglycemia for some patients. Remember, we are all different biochemically, and some patients will become symptomatic at glucose levels that other patients may tolerate well. I find that many patients who were labeled "normal" by other doctors really have a treatable condition if they could just get someone to take it seriously. How the patient responds to treatment tells us a great deal. Even the test gives us a great deal of information. If a patient becomes symptomatic at a blood glucose level of 65 mg/dL during the fourth hour of our test, this usually means that when we prevent that drop in blood sugar, by our treatment program, they will notice improvement almost immediately. Their tiredness and "brain fog" will clear, and their rapid pulse will become a thing of the past. When a patient improves dramatically with treatment, for me, it is presumptive evidence of the accuracy of this diagnosis.

What's happening here is that as the glucose level in the blood drops, the level in the brain also drops. Unlike other body tissues, such as muscle tissues, which can burn any fuel (protein, starch, sugar, or fat), the brain can only utilize or "burn" glucose for energy. If the level of glucose in the brain drops, the brain cannot function properly, leading to the neurological symptoms depicted in the above list.

The treatment of hypoglycemia is essentially threefold. Most important is the institution of a high protein, low carbohydrate diet. There are a host of these diets readily available today: Dr. Atkin's, South Beach, Protein Power, Suzanne Summers', Sugar Buster's, Dr. Schwarzbein, Dr. Shoemaker's, and others. All share the concept of high protein and low carbohydrate intake with minor variations between them. How low on carbohydrates? That depends on the individual: some patients have a fragile system and can handle only 20 gm a day, while others can tolerate between 40 and 60 gm daily. Most will need somewhere between 20 gm and 40 gm for optimal functioning. I hope that the rationale for this diet is obvious: if you don't eat carbohydrates, you don't set off the over-reacting pancreatic production of insulin, and hence the blood sugar doesn't fall as dramatically. I usually start with the Atkins diet, as patients find the instructions clear, and this diet is quite doable. As patients develop more awareness and knowledge about the relationship of their symptoms to their carbohydrate intake, they may be able to move to the less restrictive diets mentioned above.

Secondly, if patients snack on high-protein, low-carbohydrate nutrients (cheese, meats, eggs, nuts, or pork rinds) just before we know their blood sugar will drop, we can also avert the intense drop in blood sugar that sets off symptoms. For example, if the blood glucose drops at three-and-a-half hours on our test, I would advise a snack timed three hours after every meal to proactively get the jump on that dropping blood sugar.

Lastly, but not as important as dietary interventions, is the use of chromium, which has been shown to have a mild ability to stabilize blood sugar levels. I typically recommend 200 mcg of chromium picolinate twice a day.

With this program, if a patient indeed has hypoglycemia, the response to our treatment is quite rapid. Within a few days many patients report feeling better than they have in years. As I have emphasized, the response to our treatment actually clarifies the diagnosis, because if the patient does not respond to this program, we need to go back to the drawing board to understand what is causing the symptoms. For many of my patients, hypoglycemia is just a part of the problem, but an important part. If overlooked, symptoms may persist despite heroic efforts in other areas.

Hypoglycemia is no myth. It is a commonly overlooked medical condition, amenable to treatment, and worth the minor inconvenience of testing to clarify both the diagnosis and treatment.

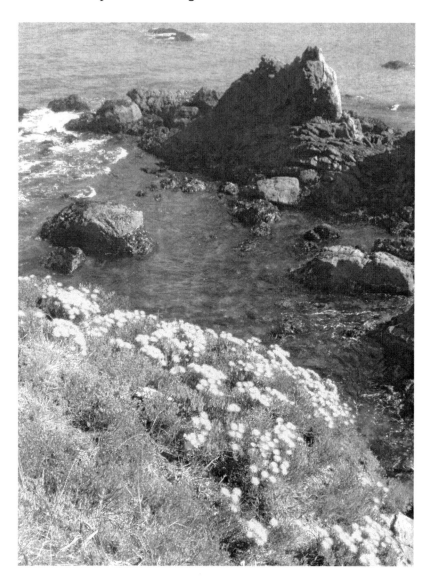

Chapter 10

Dental Contribution to Chronic Illness

The Tooth, the Whole Tooth, and Nothing but the Tooth

Why did the Zen Buddhist refuse Novocain when he needed to have his tooth pulled? Because he wanted to *transcend dental medication*. This bad but clever pun will help to launch us into a discussion of dental toxicities.

It is curious that in the field of medicine, especially for family physicians such as me, who are trained in looking at all systems of the body, somehow two areas have carved out niches for themselves that are so "specialized" that most physicians know very little about them. Those areas are podiatry (the feet) and dentistry. In all of our medical education, these areas receive short shrift, and we are encouraged to refer every problem in these areas to practitioners of those fields. Consequently, most medical doctors know precious little about the feet or the mouth, and during our medical education and training, we almost got the sense that this information was an unnecessary part of our working knowledge base. It has always seemed a bit strange to me that we have only these two subjects that we are not supposed to know enough about to direct our patients properly.

Over the years, it has become clear that there are, indeed, a number of dental problems that can greatly affect the whole body. These include mercury toxicity, electrical effects of the different metals that may be present in the mouth, metal allergy, root canal effects, and the effects of dental appliances. Let's delve into these areas, but be advised that most dentists are not aware of much of this information either. In fact, imagine the class action suits that would occur if the dental profession acknowledged that metal amalgam fillings (with a large percentage of mercury) had been harming us for years. In this medical, legal world, that won't happen. So if you attempt to discuss this with your dentist, more often than not she will tell you that these concerns are silly or trivial. However, despite that attitude, the fact is that mercury is a seriously toxic metal for the body even when it is present in only miniscule amounts.

We have known about the toxicity of mercury for many years. Calomel, a mercury-containing compound, had been used since the eighteenth century to treat a wide variety of medical conditions. When used "properly" in those times, calomel gradually made those who used it sicker and sicker, until their hair fell out and they began to salivate uncontrollably. Perversely, these symptoms were taken as a sign that the mercury was beginning to work. It was eventually, albeit slowly, recognized that mercury was truly toxic, and it was removed from the shelves as a dangerous material by the late nineteenth century.

When it was proposed in the 1930s that dental amalgams should utilize mercury as a major ingredient to more easily shape and work the filling materials, it was hotly debated for several years at the American Dental Association's annual meeting. Ultimately, it was decided that the convenience of adding mercury to other metals for the purpose of making dental fillings outweighed the risks of toxicity. So for the past seventy-five years, the public has been exposed to these dental amalgams. I would venture to say that there are very few mouths in my practice that don't have some of these metal fillings in them, with mercury as a significant component. As time has passed, we have begun to recognize that this may not have been wise. Considering that mercury thermometers are no longer available to the public because of the danger that the mercury represents, and that dentists are required by Federal agencies to dispose of their mercury as hazardous waste, it seems strange that the dental profession would be so reluctant to admit that mercury might be dangerous.

Colorado dentist Hal Huggins has devoted his life to bringing forward this information about mercury toxicity. He found that when he removed the fillings of very ill patients, many of them recovered from a

variety of medical conditions, including rheumatoid arthritis and neurological impairments like Parkinson's disease and amyotrophic lateral sclerosis (ALS). Huggins also recognized that mercury *sublimates*,
which means that it can move directly from a solid to a gaseous form,
without becoming a liquid, just like dry ice. When mercury-containing
amalgams are scraped with dental tools, significant amounts of this
mercury gas can be released into the body. It can then move directly
into body tissues, especially the brain and nerves, where it is bound
tightly and directly poisons those tissues. Huggins' pioneering work led,
unfortunately, to his persecution and the loss of his dental license in
Colorado. He has continued to practice and teach in Mexico. Fortunately, enough open-minded dentists began to heed his message and
learn his techniques, and his research has continued to grow.

While I suspect that dental amalgams are the major source of mercury
toxicity, there are other sources as well. Consumption of certain fish
can contribute to mercury toxicity, and there are published lists of
which fish are to be avoided or limited. For example, signs are posted
in the remote, pristine White Mountains of New Hampshire telling
anglers that they should limit their consumption of trout to one per
month. For over twenty years, the health department of the state of
Minnesota has published mercury levels of the different game fish in
the state, and this should be available from almost every other state
department of health as well. In the food chain, as small fish are eaten
by bigger fish, we find the highest levels of mercury in the largest
predatory fish, such as shark and swordfish.

We also come into contact with mercury in our environment. A
small amount can be inhaled by those who live in close proximity to
coal-burning plants, and it has been recently realized that the mercury
produced by the coal-burning factories in China ascends into the atmosphere and comes down onto our soil as the prevailing winds blow
east across the Pacific Ocean.

Yet another source of mercury is found in vaccinations. Since the
1930s, vaccine manufacturers have used thimerosol, a mercury-containing
preservative intended to fight off bacterial contamination. Although it
is known that young, developing brains and nervous systems are much
more sensitive to mercury and much less able to process or detoxify
it, most of our children have been exposed to toxic levels of mercury

from this source. Until recently, each thimerosol-containing vaccine has provided up to 5 parts per million (ppm) of mercury with each injection. This is the upper limit of exposure for mercury (as established by Federal standards) for a child. However, the vaccine manufacturers, along with the pediatric profession, have encouraged the "bundling" of vaccines. This entails providing not one vaccine, but a whole package of vaccines at one pediatric visit, so that a child might receive up to 125 ppm of mercury at a single visit! Many experts have come to suspect that the explosion of autism and Attention-Deficit/Hyperactivity Disorder (ADHD) may in part be linked to these vaccinations.

Several physicians prominent in this area, most notably Stephanie Cave, M.D., have published widely and spoken before Congress repeatedly, pleading that thimerosol be removed from these vaccines. In response to this call for action, fortunately, vaccine manufacturers have minimized (but not completely eliminated) the amount of thimerosol in most vaccines. Concerned parents should really check into their children's vaccinations to be sure they are safe. Flu shots, for example, still contain thimerosol, yet medical authorities now strongly encourage the use of that vaccine in small children. By countering the negative effects of mercury, pioneering physicians in the field of autism have helped many children recover or improve. This is a part of a more comprehensive treatment program for autism, which we'll discuss in more detail in Chapter 22.

Germany and Canada have discouraged the use of mercury amalgams. England has taken this problem so seriously that, several years ago, the country passed a law that requires the mercury amalgam fillings of the deceased who await cremation to be removed prior to cremation, so that mercury vapor will not be released into the atmosphere.

If you need to have a filling replaced, please do not allow your dentist to use a mercury-containing, silver-colored amalgam. There are many viable alternatives to using mercury-based fillings. However, merely switching to plastic based fillings may not be much healthier. One of the more common plastic replacement materials contains a great deal of bisphenol-A, a toxic chemical which can do just as much harm as the mercury. Should you need your fillings replaced, I would strongly advise that you look for a dentist specifically trained in this information, referred to as a *biological* or *holistic* dentist. But a word of warning: it has been my patients' experience that when they bring this up for discussion with their usual dentist, they are usually told, "There is more mercury in a can of tuna fish than there is in your mouth." Not only is this untrue, but keep in mind that when the dentist works on the fillings already present in your mouth, scraping them will release mercury vapors, which will add to whatever mercury burden is already present.

The only tool we initially had to evaluate for mercury toxicity was hair analysis. I can't count how many patients whose hair I tested with negative results. It turns out that there are several problems with hair analysis, especially when testing mercury. First, mercury tends to bind more tightly to other body tissues, so much so that if it is present in the body, we will not find it with simple tests of hair, urine, blood, or stool. That's not where it's present. Second, the results of hair analysis have always been difficult to reproduce. This means that if you cut some hair from your head, separate it into three different batches, and send those to the same laboratory, it is likely that the results will be quite different in all three specimens. This lack of reproducibility has always cast a shadow over results, and I have found the results of hair analysis to be inaccurate to the point that I don't use it anymore.

So how *do* we check for mercury toxicity? Since it binds so tightly to body tissues, what we need to do is use a chelating material to bind tighter to the mercury than your body tissues do, and then we can pull the chelated (bound) mercury out through the urine. If there is a significant amount of mercury in a patient's tissues, we will find significant amounts of mercury in his urine as well.

The procedure goes as follows: A patient receives a brief, fifteen-minute intravenous infusion with DMPS, a chemical that binds tightly to mercury. The patient then collects all of her urine for a timed period of six to twenty-four hours, and this is mailed to a laboratory that can measure toxicity of heavy metals, of which mercury is a prime example. This is an accurate and elegant test. The amount of mercury measured in the urine is a clear measure of the amount of mercury present in the body, and hence an accurate measure of the mercury toxicity present in the patient.

As a result of this testing process, we can also learn about the presence of other possible heavy metal toxins: lead, aluminum, nickel, cadmium, arsenic, and others. If we find it, we can treat it, and the removal of other heavy metal toxins may be an important part of our treatment program. While the details of this testing and treatment process may vary from one clinician to another, this discussion represents an accurate consensus. Those patients, especially children, for whom we would prefer not using an intravenous procedure to deliver the binding or chelating chemical, will benefit from an oral chelating material called DMSA. It is not as strong as DMPS in its ability to pull mercury out of the tissues, but it still allows us to perform the analysis on children safely, without being invasive.

The treatment for mercury toxicity is similar to the process of diagnosis; we can use regular, monthly intravenous infusions of DMPS or regular oral doses of DMSA to pull mercury out of the body. While for strictly chemical reasons, chelating agents are utilized for their ability to preferentially bind to the heavy metal toxins, to a small extent they will also bind to some of the essential minerals we need for health and pull them out of the body, too. Therefore, patients should supplement these treatments with oral minerals, which include trace minerals. However, minerals should not be taken on the day of or the day after chelation treatments, since we don't want to use the binding properties of the chelator to remove the good minerals, and we don't want to waste the chelation effects by binding the good minerals in lieu of the heavy metal toxins. It is also helpful to add some weaker, natural chelating materials such as vitamin C, chlorella, alpha lipoic acid, and garlic to the program. Those interested in this diagnosis and treatment should seek help from physicians trained in the chelation process. The American College of Advancement in Medicine (ACAM) and the International College of Integrative Medicine (ICIM) train physicians in the correct use of these materials, and they should be contacted for a list of physicians in your area who do this properly.

Several years ago, a forty-year-old gentleman presented to me with the sudden onset of rheumatoid arthritis. He was working in a difficult environment, several states distant from our office, and for financial reasons, he really needed to keep working at his job but could barely do so. I scrutinized his health history and could not quite understand the sudden onset of his arthritis until I asked about recent dental work. Yes, just two weeks before the onset of his arthritis, he had had extensive dental work done. When I did the DMPS test on him, not only did it show the highest mercury level of any patient we've ever measured, but he experienced marked relief of his joint pains for the next three days simply from pulling the small fraction of mercury out of his body with the DMPS chelator used in his test! Unfortunately, as he worked a long distance from our office, and because his family was not supportive of this form of treatment, he pursued more conventional methods of treatment and was lost to follow-up.

I suspect that if we could have removed all of the mercury from his body, he would have done well. It is my experience that rheumatoid arthritis and other autoimmune diseases (such as multiple sclerosis, lupus erythematosis, and scleroderma), chronic fatigue, fibromyalgia, autism, ADHD, and a variety of neurological impairments (such as Parkinson's disease, memory loss and other cognitive difficulties) are often linked to mercury toxicity. Many other physicians have made similar observations. One of the tip-offs in a patient's history that suggests that mercury may be part of the problem is the sudden onset of memory loss. A forty-three-year-old, very successful realtor presented to our office several years ago, with just such a problem.

Ed's Story

Ed was a million-dollar-a-year realtor, very sharp and focused in all of his work activities. But all of a sudden, his memory began to fail him; he couldn't think clearly or even remember his own phone number. He simultaneously developed the onset of fatigue and headaches. He was very frustrated and worried by this sudden turn of events, and visits to several physicians' offices had provided no answers. On my initial testing for Ed, along with DHEA deficiency, I found significant levels of mercury in his urine on DMPS testing. Because of his mouth full of old silver amalgam fillings, I felt his symptoms were most likely caused by mercury toxicity. So I treated him with DHEA, 50 mg each morning, and intravenous DMPS on a monthly basis. We also referred him to a biological dentist for the proper removal of his amalgam fillings. DMPS typically pulls 1 ng/DL of mercury out of the body per treatment, so the number of

*treatments usually depends simply on the initial level of mer-
cury, which we obtain at our first analysis.*

*After six months of treatment, Ed had greatly improved, and
within a year he was back at work at full capacity. Not only could
he think clearly again, but his headaches and fatigue had also
disappeared. This improvement from the treatment of mercury
toxicity is a fairly typical occurrence in our office, and it underscores the importance of looking for this diagnosis when
the appropriate symptoms are present. This is a problem with
chronic mercury toxicity of which the public is almost unaware.*

In addition to potential mercury toxicity, metal amalgam fillings
may have yet another component of toxicity: the imbalanced or abnormal electrical potential of the teeth. This jaw-breaking phrase (sorry
about the pun) actually represents a simple concept. Whenever various
metals are in close proximity, they essentially create a battery, which
produces an electrical charge. Even the same dentist working with the
same equipment does not create the same balance of metals in each
amalgam filling. Each filling, therefore, is different in terms of the
exact proportion of its metals. If you have a silver amalgam and next
to it a gold filling, or stainless steel crown, or metal found beneath the
placement for a crown, or a metallic plate or bridge, we have the presence
of multiple metals in close proximity, creating significant electrical
charges around each tooth.

The presence of these electrical charges can be readily measured.
Dentists trained in this concept can simply place a probe against each
tooth and individually measure the electrical charge. If a significant
negative charge is present, the patient essentially has a battery located
mere inches from the base of the brain. It's not much of a stretch to
think that you could, in this way, short out some of the brain's electrical
activity. Unfortunately, the majority of dentists are not yet aware of
this information, so they do not have the equipment in their office
to take these measurements. If this information seems important to
you, seek a dental professional with the knowledge and equipment to
evaluate your problem.

Ten years ago, a fifty-year-old gentleman presented to our office with severe ringing in the ears, which we call *tinnitus*. The ringing was so loud, so constant, so insistent, that he had become depressed and non-functional and was awarded disability from Social Security (which is not easy to come by these days). Worse, his depression had become so intense that he had become suicidal, as he felt he could no longer continue to live with this constant assault on his nervous system. We had him test the electrical potential of his teeth, and it showed markedly abnormal electrical charges in his largely amalgam-filled mouth. When the dentist we referred him to removed the first few amalgams, his tinnitus was markedly reduced, and by the time the fillings were completely replaced, his tinnitus was completely gone. He was a most grateful patient, but it is not likely that he would have improved had we not taken these concepts into consideration.

Another potential cause of dental toxicity is that of root canals. George Meinig, D.D.S., president of the Root Canal Society in dentistry for many years, came to the realization that he had contributed to making many of his patients sick. He wrote a most courageous book: *Root Canal Cover-Up Exposed!* Dr. Meinig had realized that when a root canal procedure is performed, the nerve to the root of the tooth is destroyed. It turns out nerves have "trophic" influences on the tissues they supply, meaning that nerves actually nourish and contribute to the blood supply of the surrounding tissues. When the nerve is killed, the blood supply of these tissues is compromised, and this makes them prone to infection. As infection sets up in these dental tissues, the toxins released from the infective agents may contribute to the patient's illness. Some of the holistic dentists who have studied this material have found remarkable improvement of health with the removal of the root canal, usually replacing it with a bridge. Since I am not a dentist and do not treat root canals, Michael Rehme, D.D.S., a holistic dentist from St. Louis, Missouri, has graciously provided me with this clinical example which we have left unedited, in the patient's own words.

Patrick's Story

I am a forty-nine-year-old doctor who was in great health. In February 2002, I went for a routine dental visit. I had no symptoms; it was a check up. X-ray films suggested that an older root canal procedure needed to be redone. An endodontist agreed, the appointment was scheduled, and then the procedure was performed. I had no problem with the procedure and felt fine after it was completed. Within two days I started to have problems. My blood pressure increased over twenty points, both systolic and diastolic. . . . Within two days of the procedure I developed right and left shoulder pain. This continued and increased over the next eight months. It affected my ability to abduct my arm—it reminded me of an earlier injury to my shoulder that I had in my early twenties. (This happened to be the same time that I had the original root canal done, but that did not make an impression until now.) The reflex for the tooth, according to the tooth chart, showed that it referred to the shoulders. Within a few days my resting pulse and my working pulse and my exercising pulse increased by about ten beats per minute. This did not improve.

As a doctor, I measure different people's grip strength. Before the root canal it averaged 220 pounds; within two days it dropped to 160 pounds. It slowly returned to 180 pounds. Shortly after the root canal, I developed a chronic athlete's foot condition over my foot reflexology point for the shoulder. Within a few months I was starting to feel some brain fog. (I was forty-nine years old!)

After reading several books on root canal problems, I knew that I had to remove the tooth, which had continued to feel non-symptomatic. . . . My dentist extracted the tooth. Within two days, my grip returned to 220 pounds, 85 percent of my shoulder pain was gone, my foot infection was gone, brain fog was gone, pulses returned to normal. . . . All of my problems were gone with the exception of the blood pressure; it is improving slower than I would like; it is getting closer to older readings. . . . I am glad that I removed the root canal tooth; I now wish that I did not wait eight months.

❖

One relatively rare cause of dental problems is that of metal allergy. An allergy to nickel, however, is not uncommon, and nickel is often used in stainless steel and other dental appliances. Occasionally, we find patients actually allergic to mercury or gold, in which case the fillings themselves may be causing an ongoing reaction that the patient cannot cure unless the fillings are removed.

One young woman I treated was a dentist who had been wrestling with chronic fatigue and fibromyalgia, and she turned out to be allergic to gold. And, of course, she had multiple gold fillings. She even noticed that when she wore gold jewelry she developed a rash and a worsening of her symptoms, but she was hesitant to admit to herself that her favorite jewelry was contributing to her illness. When we tested her blood with the ELISA/ACT test (which we referred to in Chapter 7), it was clear that gold was the problem. She reluctantly realized she would have to stop wearing her gold jewelry and get her gold fillings replaced.

Other possible dental sources that may contribute to health impairments can be found in the form of appliances placed into the mouth. I have had three patients just this year who developed the sudden onset of seizures following the tightening of newly applied braces. Other patients have had exacerbations of their headaches (especially migraines) or the sudden onset of tinnitus and ear pain when their braces were tightened or their spacers expanded. One young man, aged eighteen, was treated by his neurologist for seizures for months with poor control. This means that, despite the use of a great deal of medication, which left him numb and sleepy and made it hard for him to function, he was still having regular seizures. I treated him with osteopathic cranial manipulation to undo the effects of the tightened braces, but the seizures did not fully resolve until his braces were removed. The orthodontist who applied the braces continued to insist that it was not possible for tightening braces to cause these problems, but improvement did not occur until this problem was addressed. Interestingly, each time the braces were tightened, the seizures got worse for this patient, and indeed for all of these youngsters. We will discuss the treatment aspects of cranial manipulation in more detail in Chapter 17, but I wanted to include this concept here.

Please understand, I am not suggesting that everyone run out to have their amalgam fillings removed. This process would involve considerable expense and pain, and the inappropriate removal of amalgam fillings could make some individuals worse. If the removal of your amalgams is even a consideration, first get your mercury levels measured and have the electrical potential of your teeth checked. If these tests are negative, there is little reason to pursue the removal of your fillings.

If we do find elevated levels of mercury in an otherwise healthy individual, what does this mean? I believe that if a patient is basically healthy, her body can throw off or handle the negative effects of that toxicity. However, if that same patient gets sick, or is exposed to additional toxins or severe stress, she may become overwhelmed by this cumulative toxicity. Now her toxic level of mercury comes into play as an additional weakening factor, which may make it more difficult for her to heal. She has become not only sick, but mercury-toxic as well. For example, when my wife and I measured our own mercury levels, we discovered they were quite elevated. We both underwent DMPS intravenous therapy to remove the mercury from our bodies. We felt there was no reason to wait for something bad to happen. Preventive medicine clearly has its place, and this is one example.

You can see that the subject of dentistry is indeed important to your health. There are other new concepts, including that of cavitation and chronic dental infections, that may also contribute to health issues. It is my intention to provide helpful directions to explore, but I cannot hope to cover all of dentistry within this book. Finding a good holistic dentist may be the first step in this segment of your journey.

Further Reading

Cave, Stephanie, and Deborah Mitchell. *What Your Doctor May Not Tell You About Children's Vaccinations.* New York: Grand Central, 2001. *(This book is an updated and excellent discussion of vaccine safety and usage.)*

Huggins, Hal A. *It's All in Your Head: The Link Between Mercury Amalgams and Illness.* Garden City, NY: Avery, 1993. *(This book provides a wonderful overview of mercury fillings and toxicity.)*

International Academy of Oral Medicine and Toxicology. IAOMT, 2007. Web. 15 Nov. 2009. <http://www.iaomt.org>. *(This site includes information about biological dentistry and will help you find a knowledgeable holistic dentist in your area.)*

Meinig, George E. *Root Canal Cover-up Exposed!* Ojai, CA: Bion, 1993. *(This book includes an in-depth discussion of the problems following root canal procedures.)*

Seafood Watch. Monterey Bay Aquarium, 2008. Web. 15 Nov. 2009. <www.seafoodwatch.org>. *(This site provides comprehensive information about the mercury content of seafood and recommendations for consumption.)*

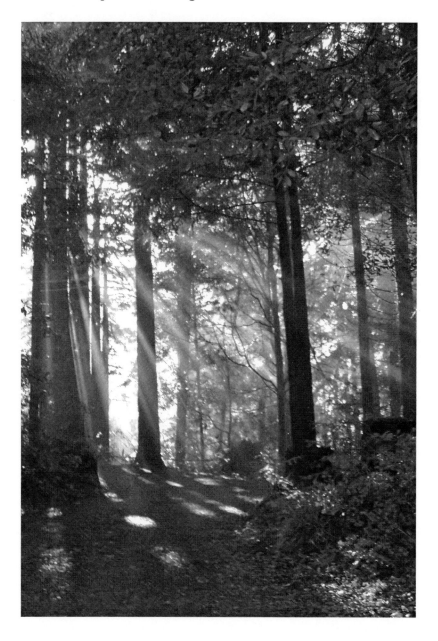

Chapter 11

Mold and Biotoxicity

There's a Fungus Among Us

When it comes to understanding the different components of chronic illness, the concept of toxicity has received a good deal of recent attention. With the publication of Dr. Ritchie Shoemaker's brilliant book *Mold Warriors*, we now have some new tools to both evaluate and treat toxicity in its different forms.

A toxin is simply a poison. Microbes in our bodies produce these poisons that make us sick, then sicker, a phenomenon referred to as *biotoxicity*. It is fairly obvious that a microbe (bacteria, virus, fungus, parasite, or other infective agent) makes us sick by infecting us, and it is equally clear that treating these disease-causing microbes will make us better. But what is just becoming clear to us is that not only do these microbes make us sick by causing an infection, but some of these microbes can, in the process of being killed by our immune system, release toxins into our bodies that make us even sicker. Because these toxins are made by microbes, which are living biological systems, we call them *biotoxins*. This term distinguishes these materials from other types of toxins such as heavy metal toxins or synthetic toxins, which are not made by living systems.

Doctors are beginning to appreciate that some of these toxins remain in the body and cannot be excreted or destroyed. Thus, they actually accumulate within our bodies. The body's natural method for processing toxins is to concentrate them in the body's main organ of detoxification: the liver. Once the biotoxins congregate in the liver, they bind to the body's bile and are sent out into the gastrointestinal tract for release in the stool. However, as the liver binds the toxin to bile and sends it into the intestines, the body's natural recycling system, which we call *enterohepatic circulation,* recirculates the bile when it reaches the small intestine. So the toxin, still attached to that bile secreted by the gall bladder, goes back to the liver rather than leaving the intestinal system, and thus accumulates within our body. Hence, even when we kill the invading microbes with our immune system, the remaining toxins continue to plague us with their harmful effects. Not everyone is subject to this problem, however. For most, the immune system recognizes these toxins and uses its defense mechanisms to destroy them. Unfortunately, about 25 percent of people are genetically unable to make an antibody to these toxins, and those patients may get progressively sicker as the toxins accumulate within their bodies.

What specific microbes are we talking about? The most common offenders are molds, especially the black mold *Stachybotrys,* but several other mold species such as *Cladosporium* and *Fusarium* can play a role in toxin formation. Harmful toxins can also be produced by certain viruses, especially those in the *Herpes* family, such as Epstein-Barr virus, which is the agent of mononucleosis; Cytomegalovirus; and Human Herpes Virus 6 (HHV-6), which is the agent of roseola infection. A new and particularly toxic strain of HHV-6 has recently been discovered and has now been linked to chronic fatigue and fibromyalgia. Lyme bacteria can also produce these toxins, as can infections with the mycoplasmas, which are infective particles between viruses and bacteria in size. The atypical pneumonias (walking pneumonia) and Gulf War syndrome are examples of these infective agents.

Dr. Shoemaker is the physician who first demonstrated the presence of toxins in our environment with his pioneering work on the *Pfiesteria* outbreak in Chesapeake Bay in 1997. He later found similar microbes in algae-borne lakes in Florida and in long-standing cases of Ciguatera poisoning (which occurs from eating certain seafood). We suspect that other microbes will be implicated as our understanding of this problem deepens.

Symptoms

So what are the symptoms of biotoxicity? Patients with this problem may experience a surprisingly wide range of symptoms related to many different organ systems. When this confusing array of symptoms is taken out of context or not understood as representing the many manifestations of biotoxicity, it is easy to see how both patients and physicians might mistakenly think that this is all "in their heads." The list below outlines these symptoms:

- Fatigue
- Muscle aches and cramps
- Unusual pains ("ice pick" or "lightning bolt")
- Sensitivity to bright light, tearing, blurred vision
- Cough, chest pain, shortness of breath
- Cognitive impairment
- Appetite swings and weight gain
- Numbness and tingling, often in unusual patterns
- Frequent urination
- Sensitivity to static electrical shocks
- Excessive thirst
- Menorrhagia (abnormal vaginal bleeding)
- Weakness
- Headaches
- Abdominal pain, nausea, diarrhea
- Chronic sinus congestion
- Joint pain with morning stiffness
- Skin sensitivity to light touch
- Mood swings
- Night sweats
- Temperature dysregulation
- Metallic taste in the mouth
- Impotence

These symptoms sound a lot like fibromyalgia or chronic fatigue or depression. In children, it might appear like ADHD. In fact, many patients with these particular diagnoses may have unrecognized biotoxicity as either a component of their illness or the direct cause, and most of them would benefit greatly from an evaluation for mold toxicity and treatment if appropriate.

Diagnosis

The first order of business is to even *consider* the diagnosis. Until I had read Dr. Shoemaker's books and studied with him, I had never thought to ask my patients about their exposure to mold or these other infective agents. Now I routinely inquire about their possible exposure to mold at home or work. Have their homes had any water damage or leakage anywhere? This includes the roof, basement, and walls. Do they notice a musty smell or see any mold? The materials that can be seen are often just the tip of the iceberg. Mold may grow inside of walls and get into the heating-cooling system of the house, sending mold spores over the entire residence. If you are wondering how this happens, be aware that sheet rock paper is made from processed tree bark, which is loaded with mold spores. To bring those spores to life, just add water. How about at work? Do co-workers have similar symptoms or complaints? As I have explored this area, it is surprising how many of my sick patients do report exposures that they had never suspected as being relevant to their illness. Keep in mind that mold toxins may remain in the body for long periods of time, so that mold exposure may have occurred in a previous residence (so I have to ask about *any* exposures) and the toxin may still be present in their body, even though they left that home several years ago.

When presented with this information, some physicians dismiss this whole subject by pointing out that in the natural world, we are literally surrounded by molds, so why are we making such a big deal out of this? It is certainly true that our natural world is filled with molds, thousands of species actually, of every shape and description. In fact, the reason that the mold species make toxins is not to damage us, but to keep other species of mold at bay as the molds try to claim their own piece of real estate in the natural world. It is a system of checks and balances, with each species holding the ones nearby at arm's (spore's) reach. However, when a species of mold can grow inside of a dampened wall with no competitors, it just grows wild and can make significantly more toxins and many more spores as it reproduces at will. While most of these species are relatively harmless to humans, several of them, including

Stachybotrys, Penicillium, Cladosporium, Fusarium and *Aspergillus*, are capable of producing a toxin that can make us quite ill. *Stachybotrys*, or black mold, is the most well-known.

Maureen's Story

Maureen was a twenty-eight-year-old woman whom I saw for the first time in March of 2006. Her symptoms had begun three years previously, when she was working in a building with a very leaky roof. She had also experienced several traumatic events at the same time, including a difficult divorce, which complicated both our evaluation and her perceptions about what may have triggered her illness. In August of 2005, Maureen began to violently throw up on a daily basis, and this went on for months. She saw multiple physicians, including several gastrointestinal specialists, and underwent extensive testing, which showed no obvious cause for her symptoms. She was diagnosed by various physicians as having bipolar disorder, irritable bowel syndrome, and hypochondriasis (meaning it was all in her head or psychosomatic). Since her initial exposure to the mold, Maureen had gained thirty-five pounds and had developed sensitivities to all sorts of chemicals and perfumes (which we call multiple chemical sensitivities). This is actually a common event following untreated biotoxin exposure. She continued to experience daily nausea and vomiting, regular headaches, and an inability to think clearly. She described her poor decision making in very simple terms: "It's like I'm inept." She also reported blurred vision and bouts of chest tightness with wheezing.

When Maureen came to me, she had just lost her job of fourteen years, at which she had been previously quite competent, and she was trying to live a normal life and raise her three children. But she could hardly function. Her energy level was very low, and she reported difficulty staying asleep and waking up un-refreshed each morning. She described joint pains in her neck, shoulders, and upper back, and she displayed the classical irritable bowel symptoms of gas, bloating, distention, and diarrhea alternating with constipation.

When I tested her vision with the Functional Acuity Contrast Test (FACT), which we will describe later, the results strongly suggested biotoxin exposure. Her DHEA test was a little low, as was her progesterone level. I started her on natural progesterone cream, ¼ tsp daily, applied to her skin. I also put her on a small dose of DHEA, and we started cholestyramine in the form of Questran Light, one scoop mixed with water three times daily, which is the best immediate treatment for mold toxicity.

When Maureen returned in April, just six weeks later, she reported that she was already 80 percent better. Her energy was markedly improved despite that fact that she was still living in her home, which had obvious mold exposure. She had a new job, was successfully working again, but noticed when she missed even a single day of her Questran, she became lethargic again. She planned to remediate her home to clean up the mold, and she was thrilled that she had her life back; she was no longer plagued by nausea, vomiting, chest pain, and joint pain.

She was so impressed with her improvement in just a short period of time, that she bought a copy of Mold Warriors to give to her family physician, who had essentially told her she was a hypochondriac. Her physician refused to even look at the book or to take Maureen's story seriously.

It has been my experience that most of our mold-toxic patients have had a similar experience to Maureen's. Their symptoms are usually misunderstood as representing psychological imbalances, particularly depression, but they do not respond well to antidepressant and anti-anxiety medications. That should be the tip-off that we need to look deeper for a cause of these symptoms. Recalling that only 25 percent of patients are genetically unable to make the antibodies they need to these toxins, these patients may live in a home with others who have no symptoms or work in a mold-laden environment where others are not sick. Family and co-workers therefore assume that since only one person is sick, that it is in his head. These patients feel like no one is listening to them, including their physicians. The trouble is that no one *is* listening. This adds even more to their burden of suffering, often tearing up families and friendships, which makes them even sicker. Now they are sick *and* depressed, but we can clearly see which came first. It is difficult to try to fight a biotoxin illness, and even more difficult when no one really believes you are sick.

The good news, however, is that we are now beginning to understand these symptoms, and there are treatments available. While no precise test exists yet for any specific toxin, we can measure the effects of toxins in several ways.

The simplest is a visual screening test called the Functional Acuity Contrast Test (FACT). This is a well-established analysis used by ophthalmologists for many years, in which the patient looks at a series of grayish lines of decreasing clarity. If the patient is unable to see the lighter lines that normal people can, this indicates poor retinal function and has been closely linked to biotoxicity. Maureen was unable to see any of the lines on the last two columns, which is strongly suggestive of biotoxin illness. If you are interested in this process, you can go to Dr. Shoemaker's website to take this test online.

Dr. Shoemaker has discovered a whole series of biochemical tests that show the patient is experiencing an inflammatory reaction to toxin. He has clearly demonstrated that a treated patient, when placed in a moldy environment, will have noticeably elevated levels of these inflammatory markers (measured in blood tests), which then come back to normal when the patient is removed from the moldy environment and treatment has been resumed. Once the diagnosis of biotoxicity has been entertained, we can begin treatment. In fact, the response to treatment confirms the diagnosis, as in Maureen's case.

Treatment

Several treatments for biotoxicity are currently in use. Dr. Shoemaker provides a combination of medications based on his testing. In its simplest form, this consists of using the binding resin cholestyramine (trade name, Questran) or its cousin, Welchol. These prescription medications are more traditionally used in the treatment of elevated cholesterol levels. But for our mold-toxic patients, these medications bind to the toxin more strongly than the toxin binds to bile, and thus the medications pull toxins out of the intestinal tract while the bile returns to the liver. This drastically decreases the body's load of toxin and allows healing to begin. Dr. Shoemaker has also discovered that combining cholestyramine with Actos provides significantly better results. Actos is usually prescribed for the treatment of diabetes, but for the treatment of mold toxicity we term this an "off-label" use. Many medications have value for the treatment of conditions other than the ones for which they are typically provided, and the "off-label" use of a medication is common in the practice of medicine.

Dr. Patricia Kane, who is an expert in the field of fatty acid metabolism, has a clinic in Philadelphia where she has put together a slightly different and more complex treatment. This consists of regular intravenous infusions of phosphatidylcholine followed by intravenous glutathione. This is combined with a special diet (similar to Dr. Shoemaker's) and many supplements. Both of the intravenous agents are natural materials that have the capacity to bind to toxins, and Dr. Kane has reported some remarkable results from her treatment.

I can confirm that for many seriously ill patients, these treatments do work, and some patients who have been given up on by their physicians as being hopeless or untreatable have been able to resume a normal life.

Barbara's Story

Barbara had been my patient for almost eight years when she came into my office in 2008 with some new and frightening symptoms. Let me provide a little medical background for Barbara's history. When I first saw Barbara, she was a thirty-four-year-old nurse who had not been able to work because of debilitating chronic fatigue, complex partial temporal lobe seizures, migraine headaches, and weakness of her right upper arm. Along with administering osteopathic cranial manipulation, which proved very helpful for her migraines and seizures, I also found her to be low in DHEA and magnesium. She had significant hypoglycemia and an overgrowth of the yeast Candida albicans and the bacterial pathogen Klebsiella. Her Lyme and heavy metal test results were negative. As I treated all of these imbalances, Barbara improved slowly and steadily, with eventual resolution of all of her symptoms. She was able to return to full-time work as a nurse. Over the next eight years, she would have occasional injuries to her neck and back that would throw her off for a few weeks, but these injuries responded well to osteopathic manipulation.

So, Barbara had essentially been quite healthy until the summer of 2008, when she appeared in my office complaining of a recurrence of her seizures, which hadn't happened in years. She was also experiencing severe migraine headaches and neck pain. With slurred speech and glazed-over eyes, she told me that she'd never felt this bad; she reported that her face felt funny and she was having strange sensations in her head. Barbara had become so weak that she could only walk with a broad-based gait, and she had developed tremors in her right hand. She also noted extreme heat intolerance and an odd sensation of chest tightness that came and went.

This sudden deterioration of cognitive and nerve function really had Barbara shaken. It had me shaken, too, as she sat before me and I watched as she could barely speak or answer questions. I immediately got an MRI scan of her brain and consulted her neurologist for evaluation. The MRI scan was clear, showing no pathology. Barbara's neurologist was unable to find a cause for these symptoms, so he prescribed her a small dose of Zoloft for depression and anxiety.

With a normal MRI result and no obvious neurological diagnosis, I started looking elsewhere for answers. We tested her vision with the FACT test and it suggested the possibility of biotoxicity. Further questioning revealed that she had noticed a funny smell in her bedroom, possibly mold, and she reported wiping some of the black mold off her window sill. The smell was similar to the mulch she had placed under the bedroom window. Only one explanation made any sense to me: with her wide array of debilitating symptoms, Barbara was suffering from biotoxicity, most likely from mold exposure. As we explored this possibility together, we discovered that the timing of this exposure fit well with the onset of her unusual symptoms. I placed her on Questran, one scoop daily and in-

creased slowly to two or more per day. She quickly started to improve, and within ten days she could think and walk again. Overall, she estimated a 50 percent improvement. Full-blown seizures were now rare, her headaches were lessening, and she could talk without difficulty. The Zoloft was clearly not helping her and only made her sleepy, so she discontinued it with my blessings.

Barbara hired an environmental consultant to check her home for mold, and it was indeed discovered under her house. Although I advised her to leave the home until it could be remediated, she was unable to do so for logistical reasons and so I added Actos, 45 mg daily, to her regimen. Within 24 hours she called me to say she was almost back to normal and was thrilled with her improvement. She admitted she had been terrified about how poorly her mind was working, and the dramatic relief that she experienced was liberating for her. The tremors and seizures had resolved and she was back to being herself again. She still has to address the mold issue, and she will need to be vigilant in the future to avoid exposures. However, Barbara now knows what she is experiencing when these symptoms reappear, and she now has the medications with which to treat them.

You can now see how devastating mold exposure can be, especially since many physicians, even experts, are unfamiliar with it as a diagnosis. It is my opinion that countless individuals suffer from this condition to different degrees. Without a clear awareness of this condition, doctors treat patients with antidepressants and other medications that might take the edge off their symptoms. These medicines, unfortunately, cannot provide the definitive help these patients so desperately need.

Keep in mind that this is *not* an infection or allergy to mold (although these can occur simultaneously, further confusing the situation). Instead, it is a reaction to mold *toxin* which, in essence, is a new concept for medical science. I have referred elsewhere to the difficulty that medicine has with embracing new concepts, and this is a perfect illustration of how the reluctance to accept new ideas can hinder a patient's ability to obtain correct diagnosis or treatment.

Further Reading

Foster, John, Patricia Kane, and Neal Speight. *The Detoxx Book.*
        BodyBio, 2002, available from www.detoxxbook.com.
Shoemaker, Ritchie C. *Mold Warriors*. Baltimore: Gateway, 2005.

Medical professions may obtain the *Functional Acuity Contrast Test (F.A.C.T.)* from Stereo Optical Company, Inc., Chicago, IL. Visit their website, www.nationaloptronics.com, or call them at (773) 867-0380.

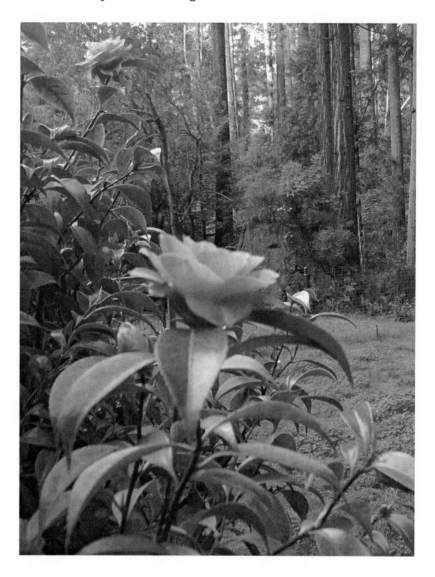

Chapter 12

Chronic Infections

Don't Bug Me Anymore!

*T*hat our universe is filled with potentially infective agents is certain. The list of infectious candidates is exhausting:

- Bacteria
- Viruses
- Rickettsia (life-forms intermediate in size between bacteria and viruses)
- Fungi and molds
- Parasites
- Prions (misfolded proteins that comprise an infectious agent)

If one were prone to paranoia, this would be an excellent place to get started. This is well illustrated in the television show *Monk*, in which actor Tony Shalhoub is so fastidious that he has difficulty shaking hands without calling immediately for his Handi Wipes. From the beginning of time, the presence of germs in our environment has been a simple reality that we've just had to accept and respect. There is nothing we can do to change it—like it or not, we share this planet with the microbes. Understandably, some anxious individuals have hoped to control or contain these organisms, but as we will see, that is not likely to be possible. On the other hand, we may not need to control them. Perhaps all we must do is find a way to coexist with them.

The good news is that our immune system is fairly well designed to do just that. When we are exposed to infectious agents, we have an elaborate method for recognizing and dealing with them. Over the eons of human evolution, we've actually developed a very complicated relationship with these organisms, some of which have been very helpful to us and continue to be so. Recent research suggests that as much as 85 percent of our DNA is actually of viral or bacterial origin! This implies that our relationship with these organisms over time has been symbiotic, or mutually beneficial. This perspective may come as a shock to those of you who assume that any infectious agent is, by definition, an enemy. I urge you to keep in mind that old aphorism: "What doesn't kill you makes you stronger."

Simple examples of this symbiotic relationship between our bodies and these organisms are plentiful. For example, the structure of our mitochondria, the little energy-making factories inside of every cell, is amazingly similar to the structure of bacteria. This suggests that somewhere in our evolution we may have co-opted these bacteria and incorporated them into our structure, making them an important part of us. Another example was given when we discussed the health of our intestines and noted that we need a good quantity and balance of beneficial bacteria, namely *Lactobacilli* and *Bifidobacteria*, for normal function. Indeed, these bacteria produce most of our vitamin B-12, so we need that relationship for our optimal functioning. Recent research goes beyond this simple co-existence between us and microbes. Evidence now suggests that the micro-organisms we were born with and acquired immediately after birth literally create a setting for our body's immune system with which we resonate for the rest of our lives. When that setting is disturbed, getting back into a balance that duplicates our original birth pattern is one key to pursuing health.

Having said this, and in trying to emphasize the biological balance that is so necessary for health, I also want to stress that certain micro-organisms, although beneficial under certain circumstances, can still create significant problems when not in proper balance with our immune system, and others are outright toxic to us.

Superbugs

The potentially serious infections are the headline grabbers. The media try to educate us about a possible future in which certain infections are potentially preeminent. Major among these infections are the *superbugs*, a term that describes what has been happening since we began using antibiotics a bit too casually. The development of penicillin in the 1940s began the discovery of a host of antibiotics that were capable of killing bacteria. Recently, we have added the ability to kill some viruses as well. This is without question one of the great achievements of modern medicine. It has allowed us, for the first time in history, to treat truly severe and life-threatening infections such as meningitis, pneumonia, and septicemia. Unfortunately, our unbridled admiration for antibiotics has led us to use them at times when they are not really necessary. For example, the majority of sinus infections, bronchitis, and ear infections are caused by viruses for which we do not yet have treatments available. There has been a huge push in the medical journals over the past five years to persuade physicians not to use an antibiotic for every one of these infections, a standard practice for the medical field. The reason for this educational effort is simple: we have slowly but surely killed off the weakest bacteria, and the stronger species have evolved biochemical mechanisms to resist our antibiotics. Thus, these bacteria get stronger and stronger with every passing decade. Some experts fear that within the next ten to twenty years, we will have very few effective antibiotics available.

Within the superbug category, the media have singled out several for our immediate attention. One is the dreaded *methicillin-resistant Staphylococcus Aureus* infection (MRSA). In fact, the S*taphylococcus* bacterium (abbreviated *Staph*) is one of the most common infectious agents. Impetigo, along with other skin infections like abscesses, wound infections, and cellulitis, as well as conditions like pneumonia, sinus infections, and ear infections, are well known to be frequently caused by *Staphylococcus*. It is against these particular bacteria that our indiscriminate use of antibiotics has surfaced with a vengeance. These bacteria are no longer susceptible to many of the antibiotics commonly in use, and we have to use several antibiotics simultaneously and for longer periods of time. When these are especially severe, we may require intravenous infusions in a hospital environment to eradicate the infection. We've already discussed in our chapter on dysbiosis how the indiscriminate use of antibiotics can kill off the good bacteria and leave more toxic bacteria and yeast behind to inflame our intestines and throw off our biochemical balance. The same effect arises from the use of antibiotics to treat any bodily system.

What we've discussed thus far is really just an overview of the problem. There are several areas that I want to cover in more detail, including some specific infections that may go unrecognized and lead to a weakened state and ultimately to the onset of chronic illness. There are aspects of these infections that are controversial, which may explain why they are often not recognized or are overlooked by many health-care providers.

Lyme Disease

There is no question that when we are bitten by ticks, *Borrelia* bacteria are injected into our bodies. Some physicians believe that this is a limited illness and that the timely use of antibiotics for ten to fourteen days will eradicate it completely and forever. This is the view of the Infectious Disease Society of America (IDSA), whose guidelines are published in the *Journal of Infectious Diseases*. They do not recognize the existence of a chronic Lyme disease, but they sometimes refer to a "post-Lyme disease syndrome." The IDSA believes that the classical bulls-eye skin rash and standard lab tests are quite reliable to make these diagnoses with precision.

Other physicians see a very different picture, and these select few have formed the International Lyme and Associated Disease Society (ILADS). These doctors, just as I, have seen thousands of patients who had seemingly prolonged illness that were direct results of Lyme infection. This chronic version of illness is much more difficult to treat than acute Lyme disease, often requiring multiple rounds of antibiotics for prolonged periods of time, sometimes intravenously. The unfortunate individuals who fall into this category of chronic Lyme disease have been weakened by their disease to such an extent that we see many of the deficiencies and imbalances alluded to earlier in this book: adrenal, thyroid, magnesium, food allergy, dysbiosis, and direct toxicities, all of them caused by both treatments and the Lyme organisms themselves.

As the patient becomes more and more depleted, we have, in essence, a biochemical domino effect in which each imbalance predisposes to the next, further depleting the patient and creating a vicious spiral downward. Ultimately this becomes so complicated that treatment for this condition has become almost an art form, and the physicians who provide this treatment are described as "Lyme literate." Some patients are so depleted that we can't even begin to give them antibiotics until we have recognized these deficiencies and built up their strength to the point where they are able to tolerate the antibiotics and respond properly. Many of these patients have negative tests for Lyme disease when they start treatment; however, these tests only measure the amount of antibodies the body has been able to create in order to counter the Lyme organism. Hence, if the immune system was weakened to the point that it could not produce these antibodies, the test would show no traces of them with our first measurements. Eventually, patients will test positive as their immune systems get stronger and treatment proceeds. We have also come to realize that when the tick injects its secretions into us, it is not just Lyme bacteria that enter our bodies: it is extremely common for the parasite *Babesia*, the bacteria *Bartonella*, and other infective agents to be injected into us at the same time! We must be aware of these co-infections so that they can be diagnosed and treated along with the Lyme organisms. Also, keep in mind that our new knowledge of biotoxicity, pioneered by Dr. Ritchie Shoemaker and discussed in our previous chapter on mold, has allowed us to understand and treat this chronic illness with a deeper understanding of its complex biochemistry. The list below illustrates some of the most common symptoms of chronic Lyme disease:

- Erythema chronicum migrans (the "bull's eye" present in 30 percent of cases)
- Recurrent joint swelling and pain
- Cardiac conduction defects (atrio-ventricular blocks, or, arrhythmias)
- Neurological symptoms:
  - Optic neuritis and atrophy
  - Cranial neuritis (Bell's palsy, affecting the 7th cranial nerve)
  - Aseptic meningitis
  - Radiculopathies (nerve root compression) especially at the cervical 5th and Thoracic 8th-12th levels
  - Cranial nerves 2, 3, and 6 effects
  - Conjunctivitis, Iritis, and Uveitis (eye inflammations)
  - Depression

- Memory loss
- Excessive daytime sleep
- Fatigue
- Extreme irritability and Emotional lability (mood swings)
- Word-finding difficulties
- Spatial disorientation
- Photo- and phono-phobia (sensitivity to light and sound)

Wow! What a complicated picture these infections can create, and with so many different symptoms that you can begin to see the problem inherent in this diagnosis. In Missouri, where this book was written, infectious disease specialists believe that we don't have much Lyme disease, so they are not inclined to diagnose or treat it. Worse, as they are the specialists in this area, this opinion has trickled down to most of the rank-and-file physicians so that they don't diagnose or treat it either. The Missouri Department of Health, however, publishes a semi-annual newsletter documenting several hundred reported cases of Lyme disease. Since Lyme disease does not require mandatory reporting by physicians, many experts believe that we really have ten to twenty times that amount of Lyme disease in our state. This represents a considerable discrepancy in opinion. As you might imagine, chronic Lyme disease is clearly under-diagnosed in Missouri, and since even acute Lyme disease is rarely diagnosed or treated, it becomes chronic, which turns it into a really difficult problem, as I've alluded to above.

Mark's Story

Mark, a cattle rancher, first came to see me six years ago, when he was forty-eight. His main concerns were diminishing energy levels, which had been bothering him for several years. He also noted the new onset of severe headaches, nausea, chest pain, and abdominal pain. He had recently been hospitalized for two weeks, and thorough testing provided no clear diagnosis other than sleep apnea. His DHEA level when we started was only at 233 ng/dL (normal is closer to 650 ng/dL). He also showed a high mercury level of 15 mcg/g creatinine on the DMPS challenge test. He had only a moderate magnesium deficiency and mild hypoglycemia. Testing for food allergy and stool analysis did not provide any useful or additional information.

Despite treating all of these components, I could only help Mark become marginally better, and he continued to wrestle with headaches, chest pain, and extreme fatigue. Symptoms fluctuated: some days he could work a full day on his ranch, and other days he could barely function. He eventually went to the Mayo Clinic, where an exhaustive analysis showed no clear cause for his symptoms.

A visual contrast test showed the likelihood of biotoxicity, so I began treatment with cholestyramine and searched for causes of his biotoxicity. Despite a negative screening test for Lyme disease and a borderline Western blot test (the only accurate test for Lyme disease), I felt that chronic Lyme disease provided the best explanation for all of his symptoms. Mark agreed to treatment with a series of antibiotics. When we added Dr. Patricia Kane's detoxification program, consisting of intravenous treatments of phosphatidylcholine and glutathione, he began to improve much more rapidly. He had several excellent responses to Christian religious healing services, but these responses did not last. Over a period of several years, slow, continued work on detoxification provided by a variety of health practitioners led to even more consistent improvement. While I cannot say with absolute certainty that Mark has been wrestling with a chronic Lyme infection, his response to treatment for that condition and his symptoms, which would be difficult to explain in any other way, lead me to believe that this is indeed his diagnosis, and he agrees.

I present Mark's case as an example of the complexity in making some of these diagnoses, but also as an example of how a hopeful, persistent approach may lead to excellent results. As of this writing, Mark is able to work long, hard hours on his cattle ranch without headaches, chest pains, or fatigue, and he now has his life back.

I fear that thousands of unfortunate patients have been suffering with the symptoms of chronic Lyme disease without realizing it. The ILADS group has noted that the classical rash of Lyme disease may be present only one-third of the time, and that the standard tests are highly inaccurate. To underscore this, in Southwest Missouri, most labs only run a screening test for Lyme disease, which is incapable of recognizing the majority of patients who have the disease. By doing this screening, which is often negative, they do not go further to conduct the more accurate Western Blot Test. And even this test can be negative in many chronically ill Lyme patients. What a mess!

Much of the unwillingness to admit that we have a serious problem of chronic Lyme disease is underscored by an intense push by the insurance industry. These companies are loath to pay for the expensive and prolonged intravenous treatments which may be necessary for a cure.

There is certainly more to say about chronic Lyme infection, but this is a start, and I can refer you to other sources for further details at the end of this chapter.

Other Bacterial Infections

Turning now to other forms of bacterial infections, I would first like to bring forth several newer concepts which may explain why, again, so much controversy surrounds our understanding of these infections.

BIOFILM

The first concept is that of biofilm. Until recently, microbiologists grew bacteria from patients' bodies in the laboratory and then tested that growth with specific antibiotics to discover which ones would work best in each patient's case. We call that test, in standard medical practice, the *culture and sensitivity test*. This nice but simplistic system postulates that each infection is caused by a single type of bacteria, which we can isolate and treat with precision. If only it were that easy.

Unfortunately, emerging evidence shows us that bacterial populations are actually mixed communities of different types of bacteria, sometimes with fungi, embedded in a matrix that it secretes around itself. We call this matrix a *biofilm*. We are learning that these complex biofilms are capable of protecting the bacteria from the various components of our immune system. To adequately treat them requires information we do not yet have—we have to be able to discern the makeup of these colonies, which will require diagnostic tools that are not yet available to most practicing clinicians. The good news is that many of these tools are under development and a brief catalogue of their names sounds like a sci-fi movie: denaturing gradient gel electrophoresis and high performance liquid chromatography, polymerase chain reaction (PCR) and pyrosequencing, along with fluorescent in-situ-hybridization.

In addition to accessing the most precise diagnostic tools, we will also need to understand the chemistry of the biofilm gel itself so we can keep it from blocking our treatments.

PANDAS

Another important set of bacterial infections that can contribute to chronic illness are the pediatric autoimmune and neurological diseases caused by Strep (PANDAS). In the past ten years, we have identified this condition in which a seemingly simple case of strep throat sets off a sudden change in behavior. This was first recognized in children but is being seen more often in adults as we have become more aware of its existence. In children, we find eating disorders, depression, anxiety, and bipolar behaviors suddenly appearing. We are also finding evidence of recent, unresolved strep infections (diagnosable with an ASO titer, a commonly available blood test, and with several more exotic tests as well). These children may respond dramatically to adequate doses of antibiotics provided over a longer-than-usual course of time. Children infected with PANDAS may also require intravenous immune globulin. Eventually, they may require a tonsillectomy for treatment, as the strep bacteria may lay dormant, or hide in the deep crypts of an infected tonsil.

CELL WALL DEFICIENT BACTERIA

A third important concept is that of *cell wall deficient bacteria*. The research demonstrating the reality of this phenomenon began in the late 1940s but never became popular, as it challenged the simplicity of the system already in place. Basically, we have learned over the years that many bacteria are capable of changing their shape and taking on the appearance of other forms as a part of their lifecycle. This means that they may look like common bacteria in one form, but even appear fungal-like in others. They can also form cysts, which for all practical purposes hide them from our immune surveillance. Going back to Lyme disease, *Borrelia* is an example of a cell wall deficient bacterium. Yet another difficulty in successfully eradicating Lyme disease is that these bacteria are capable of going into a cystic phase, making it much more difficult to reach or eliminate them with simple, short courses of antibiotics.

Several excellent textbooks have been written covering the idea of cell wall deficient bacteria. One of the more notable books is *Cell Wall Deficient Forms: Stealth Pathogens* (1993), written by noted clinical microbiologist Lida Mattman, and another slightly older text is *Cell Wall Deficient Bacteria* (1982), by Gerald Domingue. Despite the publishing of these well-documented textbooks, most microbiologists and clinicians have been slow to embrace this field of study. But we can't wait much longer. This concept may help us to better understand what we are facing in illness. We will discuss these cell wall deficient bacteria in more detail in the chapter on cancers, when we describe the pioneering research by Dr. Virginia Livingston.

COGNITIVE DISSONANCE

So far, doesn't this model of microbiology sound similar to our chronic disease model? It should. We are seeing the results of trying to simplify something that is really complicated, and, in the process of oversimplification, we are limiting our vision, our scope of treatments, and our possibilities for diagnosis. We refer to this psychological process underlying our oversimplification as *cognitive dissonance*. This phrase describes what we do with new information that doesn't fit into nice, neat little categories in our mind. If new information is received, if it has no box or category to fit into, we discard the information entirely, sometimes doubting its very existence. We don't want to be faced with the struggle of having to change our mind about it or deal with it. We've seen this phenomenon before in our discussions of chronic *Candida* infections, hypoglycemia, food allergy, Wilson's syndrome, and now Lyme disease. We will see it again very soon when we discuss chronic Epstein-Barr and other viral infections.

These illnesses, if accepted in their full complexity, are much more difficult to treat than a sore throat or bladder infection. Unfortunately, they are not rare, and these problems won't go away just because they require more time and attention. Cognitive dissonance allows us to deny their existence, but that doesn't change their reality or impact.

If a physician is uncomfortable with a complicated treatment, that's fine. No doctor should be asked to leave her own comfort zone. But a physician should at least *acknowledge* the complexity of this material and not deny its existence. This only leaves the patient to wonder at his own sanity, which, alas, is often the result.

Is what I am discussing complicated? You bet it is. And controversial, too. That is just its nature. I believe we have enough knowledge now that we can begin the process of dealing with this complicated material in a useful and therapeutic manner. And that's what I'm trying to do in this book.

VIRAL INFECTIONS

Bacteria are single-celled organisms with a nucleus and a cell membrane. They, like all cells, have to metabolize, make new structures, obtain nutrients, remove wastes, and "breathe" in one form or another. Viruses, on the other hand, are a different critter entirely. They consist of a core of genetic material, either RNA or DNA, so that the virus can replicate itself, and the viruses are wrapped in a coat of protein. A virus doesn't have a nucleus, really, nor does it need to "breathe" or carry out other typical functions of cells. It isn't clear if it is really alive or not, since all it does is reproduce itself, which we experience as an invasion of our body.

Once again, it is our intact immune system that allows us to recognize the foreign nature of the virus and fight it off. Usually it does so relatively easily, and the majority of viral infections, when they are eradicated, are gone. We may have even developed long-lasting immunity to that virus. However, there is a whole family of viruses which are uniquely difficult for us to deal with. They are the herpes viruses, and we number them from 1 to 8, each with a different name and slightly different focus of infection. Table 12.1 illustrates these types and their common traits.

Most of us are familiar with many of these viral strains. What the members of this family have in common is the ability to *hide* from our immune system so that we don't completely recognize or eradicate it. In fact, new research shows us that these viruses actually have methods for altering the structure of their DNA to facilitate this hiding process. What we have known for quite some time is that when the virus feels threatened by our immune system, it can move deep into our nerve cells and wait until the immune surveillance goes away. The most obvious example of this is shingles, in which the virus goes directly into the nerve ganglions and specifically infects nerve tissue. Sometimes the virus lingers, causing a rather severe pain called *postherpetic neuralgia*.

Years ago, when chronic fatigue syndrome first began to appear, it

Herpes Virus species	Common Abbreviation	Diseases Caused by Virus
Herpes simplex virus-1	HSV-1	Oral herpes
Herpes simplex virus-2	HSV-2	Genital herpes
Varicella-Zoster virus	VZV	Chicken pox, shingles
Epstein-Barr virus	EBV	Mononucleosis
Cytomegalovirus	CMV	"Mono-like" flu
Human herpes virus-6	HHV-6	Roseola, MS, fatigue
Human herpes virus-7	HHV-7	Pityriasis rosea
Human herpes virus-8	HHV-8	Kaposi's sarcoma

Table 12.1 Herpes Family of Viruses

was proposed that chronic Epstein-Barr virus (EBV) was a cause. An excellent paper by Dr. Jay Goldstein, who pioneered some of the early understanding and treatment of chronic fatigue, provided evidence for this connection. Unfortunately, EBV is a common infection, and conventional medicine dismissed it as an irrelevant cause of chronic illness since "everyone" had it. It was also true at that time that we physicians had little to nothing to offer in the way of treatment, so this component of chronic fatigue lay neglected.

Several recent developments have spurred our interest in chronic viral infections as a component of chronic illness. One is new research by Dr. Jose Montoya, an infectious disease specialist from Stanford University. He administered large doses of antiviral antibiotics (Valcyte and Valtrex) to afflicted patients for six months, and these medications initially showed significant improvement in patients with chronic fatigue syndrome who tested positive to Human Herpesvirus 6 (HHV-6) and EBV. Unfortunately, those benefits did not hold, but the research gives us hope that successful treatments may be just around the corner. While it is true that most people test positive for exposure to these viruses, those with chronic fatigue have significantly higher viral titers on blood tests, and newer methods of detection for these viruses are more accurate. Our detection methods are still nowhere near as accurate as we need them to be, but it's a start.

More recently, a unique treatment for these viruses was developed by Dr. Joe Brewer, an infectious disease specialist in Kansas City. Brewer created a "transfer factor" specific for each virus he wanted to treat. That is, since cows do not get these specific viral infections, he injected purified forms of several (HHV-6, CMV, EBV, and herpes viruses 1, 2, and 3) into pregnant cows' udders, so that they made antibodies to each virus. He purified the antibody into a form called a *transfer factor*, which is now available for oral use from several different companies. He discovered that if the patients took the transfer factor for six months, some of them got well but soon relapsed. If they took it for a year, 40 percent were cured. After eighteen months, 60 percent were cured. And the longer the product was used, the less the chance of relapse. For the first time, true cures of these chronic viral illnesses were possible. Even though a complete cure takes longer, those who respond usually note marked improvement after four months.

Kendra's Story

Thirty-five-year-old Kendra came to my office with a history of sporadic fatigue and cognitive difficulties, along with episodes of asthma. She had already been treated previously for mercury toxicity and had responded well to chelation treatments. Her DHEA level was low at 192 ng/dL, (normal for her age should have been around 650 ng/dL), so I provided DHEA supplementation, and I also treated her food allergies. These led to modest benefits, until we discovered an elevated EBV viral titer (a blood test showing antibodies to EBV virus and quantifying it) and began her on transfer factor therapy specific for EBV virus.

When Kendra began taking the transfer factors, she became much more fatigued and had a recurrence of most of her symptoms. While this is of concern, it is not unusual and actually confirms EBV as a significant component of her illness. If it wasn't, she would have had no reaction to the transfer factors at all. So we decreased the starting dose, and she cut back on the frequency of taking it to every third day until she was able to tolerate the transfer factors with no side effects. Slowly but steadily, over several months, she was able to work up to the full dose of supplement, and by the fourth month reported marked improvement in all of her symptoms. At that point, she discovered that if she missed a few doses, symptoms would return, only to disappear when she took them more faithfully. Kendra was able to discontinue the transfer factors after eighteen months and her progress held steady.

MYCOBACTERIA

In between the size of a viral particle and a bacterium are the organisms we call *mycobacteria*. The most common illness caused by an infection of these organisms is "walking pneumonia," also called *atypical pneumonia*.

We have also recognized that Gulf War illness, another severe, chronic illness largely ignored or denied by the medical profession, was strongly associated with some unusual mycobacterial infections. This connection was expressed in work pioneered by Garth Nicholson, the President and Chief Scientific Officer at the Institute of Molecular Medicine, in South Laguna Beach, California. We have learned over time that many of our Gulf War returnees needed to be treated with an average of six rounds of antibiotics, lasting six weeks each, to achieve a complete cure. Many chronic illnesses have been linked to these infections, including amyotrophic lateral sclerosis (ALS, or Lou Gehrig's disease) and chronic fatigue.

Once again, as we explore these concepts, we have hope. When a teenager or young adult presents to me with chronic fatigue and fibromyalgia, unfortunately an increasingly common occurrence in my practice, usually we find EBV infection, even if she was never formally diagnosed with mononucleosis. By the time I see her, often several years have elapsed, and as her body has weakened, we find a depleted adrenal and thyroid function. By treating these three areas, many patients recover completely within just a few months. It is inspiring to see youngsters who have had their lives so limited by illness resume their lives whole-heartedly.

Hallie's Story

Hallie first came to my office five years ago, when she was twenty-eight years old. She had been diagnosed by a rheumatologist as having fibromyalgia and was told she should just grow up and live with it. Her symptoms began six years before, when she was involved in a motor vehicle accident and sustained injuries to her neck and upper shoulder. As time went on, she got worse and the joint pain increased and spread to other areas. It is not unusual for an injury to progress to full-blown fibromyalgia, as it did for Hallie.

I began treating her with osteopathic manipulation (see Chapter 17) for her neck and shoulder areas, and discovered a low DHEA level of 110 ng/dL (for her age, it should have been about 800 ng/dL). I also noted a low magnesium level of 31.2 mEq/L (the normal range is 33.9 to 41.0 mEq/L). We supplemented her with DHEA at a dose of 50 mg each morning and provided magnesium taurate in 125 mg capsules, two at bedtime. After several months of treatment, she was somewhat better, but we were still trying to achieve complete healing. As I have just described, when really young people get chronic fatigue and fibromyalgia, most of them turn out to have had an EBV infection, even if they were unaware of having mononucleosis as a teenager. So we then measured her Epstein-Barr viral levels and the lab reported them to be extremely high. I prescribed transfer factors for her, and within several months she returned to our office describing marked improvement in all areas. She continued her transfer factors for several years, telling us she was "almost" well. We continued our diagnostic exploration, and after making the additional diagnoses of a chronic Candida infection and low cortisol, both of which were treated, she completed the final stages of her healing journey, with complete relief from her symptoms of fibromyalgia and chronic fatigue.

Of our various interventions, Hallie considered taking the transfer factors for her EBV infection as providing the most impressive results. She had no memory of having had mononucleosis as a teenager, and this is not unusual in our practice. This case emphasizes that when a youngster comes to me with a history of not feeling well since high school, this is often a tip-off that we need to look for residual, chronic EBV infection and treat it. The good news is that now we can.

Further Reading

Goldstein, Jay A. *Betrayal by the Brain: The Neurologic Basis of Chronic Fatigue Syndrome, Fibromyalgia Syndrome and Related Neural Network Disorders*. New York: Routledge, 1996.

CALDA, the California Lyme Disease Association, publishes a quarterly journal called the *Lyme Times*, www.lymedisease.org. ILADS can be accessed through www.ilads.org.

¯For transfer factor information and availability (with emphasis on EB Broad Spectrum and H6 Broad Spectrum), see researchednutritionals.com.

Chapter 13

Amino Acids and Neurotransmitters

This Is Getting on My Nerves

The word *neurotransmitter* sounds imposing, but it simply refers to those natural chemicals that assist in the transmission of electrical impulses through our nerves (neurons). When the electrical impulse that fires through every nerve in our body reaches the outer cellular limit of a neuron, or nerve cell, the energy of that impulse is translated into a chemical reaction. Those chemicals involved in these reactions are our neurotransmitters. These neurotransmitters then cross the microscopic gap between nerves, called a *synapse*. When the chemical reaches the other side of the synapse, it again is translated into a fired-up electrical impulse, and the communication process continues. Dozens of neurotransmitter chemicals are known, but several are considered of overriding importance to our health.

The best known of these neurotransmitters is probably *serotonin*, which plays a central role in preventing depression, controlling pain, and allowing sleep. Almost everyone is familiar with the anti-depressant medications widely advertised on television: Zoloft, Prozac, Paxil, Effexor, Celexa, Lexapro, and Cymbalta. All of these belong to the family of antidepressants we call *specific serotonin reuptake inhibitors* (SSRIs). While the full name is a mouthful, it accurately reflects what these medications do. When the chemical, in this case serotonin, reaches its destination at the end of the synapse, it has completed its job. The serotonin is then normally broken down by enzymes, so that more serotonin can be released from the other end of the neuron, and the process can continue. If we slow down or inhibit this enzymatic process by using SSRIs, we artificially increase the amount of serotonin available in the synapse and the brain gets the impression that it has all of the serotonin it needs. As the name suggests, the reuptake of serotonin is thus inhibited. What most physicians seem to ignore is that this artificially created sense that we have an adequate level of serotonin will eventually send a message to the brain that it is doing fine, and that we don't have to keep making more. So the chemical process by which serotonin is made basically takes a vacation and what we see, clinically, is that patients on these medications need to take more and more of their medication to get the same effect or switch medications when, eventually, this same process is repeated. Wouldn't it make more sense to give the body the raw materials by which it could manufacture more of what it needs? Yes, it would, and this is actually possible.

Several physicians, including Marty Hinz and Tom Urcini at Neuro Research in Duluth, Minnesota, have been studying this problem for the last fifteen years. While their focus has been primarily on obesity, which they see as a major neurotransmitter deficiency disease, they have also observed that a wide variety of medical problems, including fibromyalgia, chronic fatigue, depression, anxiety, anorexia, bulimia, panic attacks, migraine headaches, Parkinson's disease, PMS, obsessive-compulsive disorder, IBS, and Crohn's disease, also seem to have neurotransmitter deficiency as an important feature.

Using a computer model with hundreds of thousands of clinical results, Hinz and Urcini have put together combinations of amino acids in specific proportions, each designed to stimulate the body to improve its production of the key neurotransmitters. The focus of their research is not only on serotonin, which we've been discussing, but also on dopamine, which in turn is made into epinephrine and norepinephrine. These four neurotransmitters, which they call the master neurotransmitters, are the focus of this innovative treatment program. Although I don't want to overwhelm the reader, I have included a diagram of the basic chemistry of the synthesis of these neurotransmitters in Figure 13.1. What I hope you can see at a glance is that the process of converting

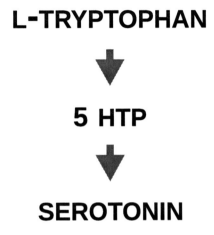

Figure 13.1   Amino Acid Basic Metabolism

these amino acids into our key neurotransmitters is a relatively simple one, involving only, one or two steps in each case. That is the main idea I would like to convey in these diagrams. For those who wish to look at this chemistry in more detail, you can see that the amino acid tryptophan is converted into 5-hydroxy-tryptophan (5HTP), which in turn is converted into serotonin. See, it's not that complicated. Figure 13.2 shows the equally straightforward process of converting the amino acid tyrosine into DOPA, which in turn is converted into dopamine and then into norepinephrine and then into epinephrine. I hope you can see that these chemical conversions are actually fairly simple.

Hinz and Ursini have discovered that by providing patients 5HTP and Tyrosine, which we call the *precursors* for neurotransmitters (because they are necessary for their synthesis and directly converted into them) in carefully orchestrated doses, unique for each patient, the body can make what it needs. These materials are provided as oral supplements, and by adding the amino acid cysteine and several co-factors that nourish these reactions also as oral supplements, they can indeed get the body

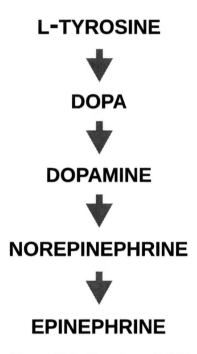

Figure 13.2   Tyrosine to DOPA

to make more of the required neurotransmitters. They report remarkable success in treating all of the conditions noted above, and I can confirm from my own experience that this is true.

Katy's Story

Katy first came to see me in 1997, when she was forty-one years old. A year and a half prior, she had been diagnosed by an ENT specialist as having temporal mandibular joint dysfunction (TMJ) and had recently been referred to an oral surgeon. TMJ is the common designation for jaw pain accompanied by clicking and popping in the jaw joints, a sense that the teeth are not properly aligned when the jaw closes, and an inability to open the jaw adequately or chew down on hard foods. Uncertain that surgery was necessary, Katy was referred to me by a colleague for osteopathic cranial manipulation. She began to respond immediately to treatment, and within a few months could chew on apples again, and within four months was essentially well. She noted that for the first time in years her jaw no longer popped. Although this part of the story is a digression on my part, and probably not related to what happened next, it does present an opportunity to give another example of the potential benefits of cranial manipulation. I continue to follow Katy and she has never required the skills of an oral surgeon.

Several years later, Katy came to me with acute hip and knee pain, which slowly progressed into pains over much of her body. Within a year, in April 2000, this condition was formally diagnosed as fibromyalgia. It was one of the worst cases of fibromyalgia I've ever seen, a diagnosis and degree of severity confirmed by several rheumatologists. She was unable to continue working at her job. She is one of the few patients for whom I had to provide large doses of pain medication and muscle relaxants for years, until she finally improved. It was a very long and arduous journey. Her muscles went into spasms so intense that they were rock-hard and palpable for days at a time. Extensive osteopathic treatments could only relieve the pain and spasms for short periods of time. Our usual evaluation and treatment, all documented with laboratory testing, helped only briefly. I looked at and treated her adrenal and thyroid deficiencies (thyroiditis confirmed), mercury toxicity, mycoplasma infection, perimenopausal hormonal deficiencies, EBV infection, Candida and bacterial pathogens, and fatty acid imbalances. None of the treatments for these deficiencies did much to bring Katy out of her compromised state. More unusual treatments, such as the use of colostrum, penicillamine, cholestyramine, and low-dose Naltrexone also had no effect. Her weight fluctuated wildly with fifty-pound swings that were baffling to both of us.

A year after her symptoms began, Katy also developed unusual paresthesias, which are sensations of numbness and tingling, over her facial areas and extremities. Neurologists had no diagnosis to offer, but after quite a bit of experimenting I found *that the medication Topamax would at least bring these symptoms under control. Consultations at Mayo Clinic and elsewhere were confusing, contradictory, and generally unhelpful. Her gall-bladder, filled with small stones, was removed in 2003, with no additional benefits to her whole system.*

Approximately six years into Katy's illness and still tread-ing water, I began the amino acid protocol, providing her with 5HTP and Tyrosine so that her body could make more of the essential neurotransmitters. Within a month, she was 50 per-cent better, and over the last few years she has continued to improve significantly. A year ago she was able to return to full-time employment in an executive position, and she has really enjoyed getting her life back. She is not completely well yet, but with the addition of the methylation protocol (which we will discuss in our next chapter), slowly and surely the symptoms are disappearing, so that she is now 75 to 80 per-cent better. I have repeatedly commended Katy for hanging in there with me as we attempted to figure out which imbalances were contributing to her illness. And, as she pointed out to me, "What choice did I have?" This is an excellent example of how, as our knowledge expands, we are able to provide effective treatments today that didn't exist eight years ago, when Katy and I started on our journey. The profound improvement provided by the amino acid treatment protocol clearly initiated her return to health.

Hinz and Ursini believe that the need for increased amounts of neurotransmitters comes from damage to the nerves themselves. They further note that neurotoxins, heavy metal toxicity, and even food reac-tions (all of which we have described as important to the understanding of chronic illness) deplete and compromise the ability of these nerves to function. The prolonged use of medications, especially anti-depressants, amphetamines, migraine medications, ephedra, caffeine, nicotine, and alcohol, further compromises the body's ability to make and sustain neurotransmitter production.

While I agree with this portion of their hypothesis, Hinz and Ursini also believe that once the amino acids have started working, they have to be taken for prolonged periods of time because the nerves have been permanently damaged. That has not been my observation. Nerves can, and do, heal. I have repeatedly noticed that when you add to the improvement in neurotransmitter function the concepts of detoxification, hormonal rebalance, treatment of occult infections, general improvement of immune function, and restoration of overall hormonal balance, most patients can maintain their own state of health once it has been restored. They do not seem to need these amino acids for long stretches of time.

I do find it useful to add these amino acids to all patients who have been on antidepressants for long periods of time, and to consider their use in all chronic illness. The amino acids have also been uniquely helpful for patients with Parkinson's disease, where these same principles apply. As we have seen in depression, where the continuing use of antidepressants depletes the body's supply of neurotransmitters, we know, too, that prolonged use of medication for Parkinson's disease, which is standard medical therapy, is also associated with a gradual weakening effect of those medications over time. This means that treatment dosages need to be steadily increased and additional medications added to continue benefits of therapy. The use of specific amino acid therapy for these patients has enabled us to lessen the amount of medication and to see improved effects of the medication already in use, over time.

Bernice's Story

I first saw Bernice when she was sixty-one years old. She had developed Parkinson's disease three years prior and had tried a variety of alternative treatments. These included the treatment for mercury toxicity and the regular use of intravenous glutathione, working up to doses of 2500 mg given three times per week. Although she did fairly well with these treatments, her tremors and difficulty with walking and movement slowly worsened and it became more and more difficult for her to function.

She was quite holistically inclined but eventually accepted a trial of conventional medication along with her alternative program. She was initially given the medication Requip, and later, following consultation with a neurologist, was switched to Sinemet 25/100, given three times daily. The improvement with conventional medication was dramatic: Bernice was able to move with considerable ease and found that her tremors had decreased significantly. Over time, however, as is often the case, the benefits of medication did not hold, and higher and higher doses of medication were required to produce the same benefits.

Unfortunately, the side effects of the higher dosage of medication were becoming more difficult for Bernice to tolerate. So we began the amino acid protocol, using the supplements called D5 and Cysreplete in small doses. (These materials simply consist of the amino acids Tyrosine and 5HTP in specific proportions, along with cysteine and several other vitamins and minerals. We start with tiny doses of each, and slowly increase the dose on a weekly schedule until we optimize our results. If we see improvement and feel that we can do even better, we can provide urine testing of the neurotransmitters to "tweak" our prescription of the amino acids and for about 20 percent of our patients, this is a helpful addition to the program. As these amino acids are natural supplements, we see very few side effects, even at high doses.)

Within a few weeks on this protocol, Bernice was able to decrease her medication to her initial levels and was clinically even better, with virtually no tremors and a smooth walking gait. She told me that the amino acids definitely agreed with her. There was no doubt that the amino acids extended the benefits of her Parkinson medication appreciably. Over the last three years, these benefits have continued unabated, and Bernice remains delighted with her improvements.

As you can see, the depletion of neurotransmitters is a common component of many chronic illnesses, and by understanding and using the appropriate amino acids, we can greatly improve this aspect of health care for our patients.

Further Reading

Braverman, Eric. *The Edge Effect: Achieve Total Health and Longevity with the Balanced Brain Advantage.* New York: Sterling, 2005. *(This book provides a detailed description of the different neurotransmitters and how they can be rebuilt by the use of natural supplements. Dr. Braverman provides some nice written tests which may help an individual to discover which neurotransmitters may be out of balance.)*

For doctors, CHK Nutrition's Web site provides a host of neurotransmitter treatment materials. You can browse their products online at NeuroReplete.com or call them at (877) 626-2220.

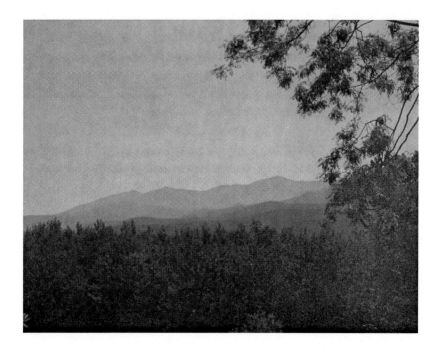

Chapter 14

Methylation: A Key to Understanding Chronic Illness

Got Methylation?

*A*s our understanding of chronic illness unfolds, it is becoming clearer that difficulties with methylation chemistry play key roles. Since even the words *methylation chemistry* are, at first glance, intimidating, let's immediately plunge into this arena. Please bear with me, since this subject is of great importance, and I hope to simplify this complex area so that we can understand how to better diagnose imbalances in these essential chemical reactions and discover what it is that we need to do to enable these reactions to work better.

The word *methylation* refers to the process of adding a methyl "group" to another molecule. A methyl group is simply composed of a carbon atom (C) surrounded by, or bound to, three hydrogen atoms (H), with one free "bond" area left. This is shown in Figure 14.1 below.

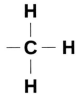

Figure 14.1 Methyl Group Illustration

These four atoms act as a unit, and moving this unit around by adding it or subtracting it from other chemical molecules is what we define as *methylation*. The importance of this unit is that it is bio-chemically essential to some very important processes in the body: namely, detoxification, the creation of energy, quenching free radicals, and repairing and restoring damaged DNA. It turns out, actually, that hundreds of chemical reactions in the body require the normal functioning of this methyl group give-and-take for us to be healthy.

So, let's say that we've taken this methyl group and placed it appropriately where it needs to go. What then? Well, then we have to make *more* methyl groups, since this is an ongoing and vital process for the body. Since what follows now consists of a fair degree of biochemical sophistication, if you'd like, you can skip ahead to less intimidating information. On the other hand, if you can pluck up a little courage, I would like to try to walk you through this material. If you can understand even pieces of this information, it will allow this whole area to make a lot more sense, and you will better understand our therapeutic strategies.

To plunge into this biochemistry, we start with the amino acid methionine, to which the body adds another methyl group to create SAM (or SAMe, chemical shorthand for S-adenosyl methionine). SAM is a critically important methyl *donor*, or contributor, so that whenever the body needs methyl groups, it calls on that molecule to provide them. Once SAM has given up its methyl group, it becomes, or, turns into SAH, which is short for S-adenosyl homocysteine, which in turn has to be converted back into methionine by several more steps, so that this whole process can continue. Figure 14.2 illustrates this process.

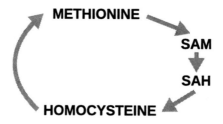

Figure 14.2   Basic Methylation Cycle to Create SAMe

That wasn't too painful, was it? Despite the long chemical names, the basic process here is simply a recycling of one molecule into another. As long as this cycle can continue functioning unimpeded, life is good. But if the body cannot keep moving this cycle along properly, homocysteine or SAH may build up, and this creates a serious problem. We have known for many years now that an excess of homocysteine is inflammatory to the body and is associated with atherosclerosis (the buildup of plaque in our arteries) and other out-of-control inflammatory processes.

For this cycle to function properly, another cycle that interfaces with this one has to work in tandem. To convert or change homocysteine back into methionine, we need adequate amounts of an enzyme, methionine synthase (MS) and that enzyme requires adequate amounts of vitamin B-12 and a derivative of folic acid, 5-CH3THF (short for 5-methyl tetrahydrofolate) to do so. Combining these cycles as they interface looks like Figure 14.3 below.

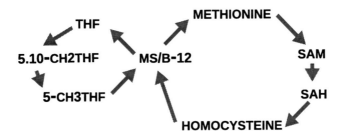

Figure 14.3   How the Folic Acid Cycle Interfaces with the Basic Methylation Cycle

Please hang tight; we're almost done with this chemistry lesson. Without focusing on the details of these cycles, you can see that they fit together like gears, and that each of these gears has to mesh properly with the others for the cycles to function properly.

The next crucial part of this chemistry is what the body *does* with homocysteine when it can't or doesn't re-make methionine, which is depicted in Figure 14.4.

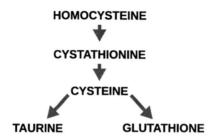

Figure 14.4   Glutathione Is Produced from the Methylation Cycle

Depending on its needs, the body makes either glutathione or taurine. Glutathione is a critical material for the body and is central for detoxification and a host of other essential chemical reactions that cannot occur without it. Taurine, on the other hand, moves these reactions into another sphere, called the transulfuration pathway, and hence we lose the opportunity to make more glutathione, which is so important for us.

Believe it or not, what I have presented thus far is a gross oversimplification of this process. The point of going into this detail is to share my excitement about some newly learned information that allows us to identify exactly where these chemical reactions are blocked up, or stuck, and use this information to provide us with natural treatments that can repair these imbalances and move these reactions into more normal alignment toward health.

Hopefully, now you can understand the basic concept of methylation and some of the basic chemistry that underlies it. With this understanding, let us review the historical background that led us to this area of study.

Although we have long known that methylation is a vital biochemical process, affecting every cell in the body, its key importance in understanding many chronic medical conditions is a rather new concept. Working with what are called *neurodegenerative diseases*, such as Parkinson's disease, Alzheimer's dementia, and multiple sclerosis, in the late 1990s, Dr. Amy Yasko from Bethel, Maine, began to make some breakthroughs with her superb understanding of methylation chemistry. When presented with the opportunity to treat an autistic child, Amy applied her technology and understanding with surprising results, and this led to many years of success with helping autistic children to heal. She speculated that other conditions, including fibromyalgia and chronic fatigue, might be biochemically related.

In 2003, a biochemist named Rich van Konynenburg picked up on this idea and showed that if you analyzed all of the known biochemical disruptions of fibromyalgia and chronic fatigue, virtually every component could be explained by difficulties with methylation chemistry.

I first heard Rich present this hypothesis at a medical meeting in August of 2007, and I was so intrigued with the logic and simplicity of his ideas that when I got home from the meeting, I immediately placed fifty-one patients with fibromyalgia and chronic fatigue on the five supplements that Rich extracted from Amy Yasko's work and described as a "Simplified Methylation Protocol." Essentially, these five materials consist of several forms of vitamin B-12 and several forms of folic acid (another vitamin in the B family). After several months of taking these supplements, I found that 70 percent of my patients had improved, and of those who improved, 20 percent were *much* better. These results were so obviously important that we proposed a research project (which was graciously funded by the Ratna Ling Study Group), to study the science of methylation in these patients and learn more about what we were doing.

Since the original fifty-one patients had already received these supplements, I offered these supplements to thirty new patients, all of whom had fibromyalgia and chronic fatigue. All of these patients had had some success with our treatment program described in this book, noting 30-70 percent improvement with their symptoms. While delighted with this improvement, all of them were still hopeful that they could do even better with additional treatments. So, all of them had gotten better and were understandably not yet satisfied with what we had achieved. We were going to look at their methylation chemistry and genetics before we started, and then have them take these supplements for six months. During this time, we would remeasure their methylation chemistry results at three months and then six months, and compare their progress with their chemistry laboratory testing. These results are hot off the presses, and I am privileged to have been able to present this research at the annual scientific meeting for the American Academy of Environmental Medicine in October 2009.

First of all, not a single patient had normal methylation chemistry to start with, and all had abnormal methylation genetics, which was measured in Dr. Yasko's laboratory.

When we looked at their initial laboratory work, done by Vitamin Diagnostics in Cliffwood Beach, New Jersey, the majority started with a low glutathione level (25 of 30 patients, or 83 percent, were low). The actual levels, which normally range from 3.8-5.5 micromol/L averaged 3.2 micromol/L in our patients. After three months, 29 of 30 patients had improved their glutathione levels (97 percent) to an average of 3.8 micromol/L.

SAM, which we have explained is of critical importance in methylation as the main methyl donor, was low initially in 20 of 30 patients, and improved in 27 of our 30 patients, which represents an increase of 90 percent in just 3 months! (See Figure 14.5.)

By the end of six months, these numbers had continued to improve, significantly. By this time, the glutathione had risen to an average of 4.3 micromol/L (remember, their starting average was 3.2, an improvement of 34 percent in that crucial metabolite). The SAM had risen to an aver-

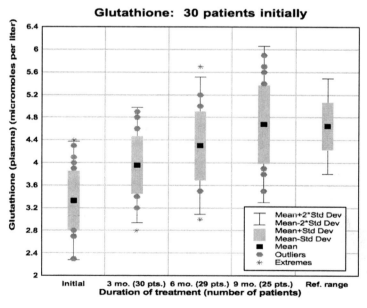

Figure 14.5   Improvement in Glutathione Levels with Methylation Protocol

age of 238 micromol/dL (from a starting level of 217 micromol/dL, an improvement of 10 percent). To put this in a different perspective, when we started, 25 of our 30 patients were low in glutathione, and 20 of 30 were low in SAM. At the completion of 6 months, only 5 patients were low in glutathione (only one patient failed to improve their glutathione level) and only 4 were low in SAM. The other methylation chemistry measures, including folic acid and folinic acid, all improved dramatically.

This is all well and good, but did these patients *feel* any better? At the start of our project, we asked all of our patients to rate, on a scale of 10, five main areas: their energy, sleep, mental clarity, pain, and overall sense of well-being. (See Figure 14.6 through Figure 14.9.)

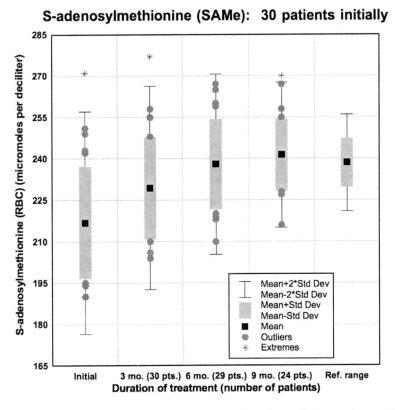

Figure 14.6 Improvement in SAMe Levels with Methylation Protocol

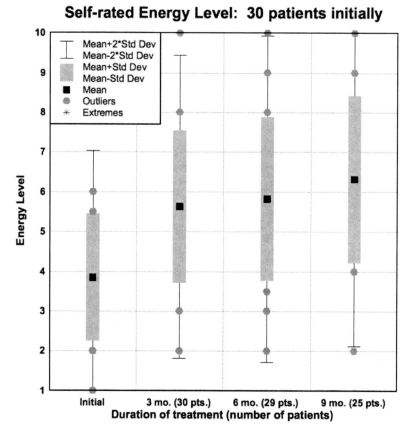

Figure 14.7   Improvement in Energy with Methylation Protocol

After three months, again they rated these areas, with improvement in energy in 77 percent of patients, improvement in sleep of 65 percent, improvement in mental clarity of 73 percent, decrease in pain in 54 percent, and an overall sense of improvement in 70 percent. These gains held up nicely at the 6 month evaluation.

From a different perspective, 83 percent told us they were improved (meaning 15-50 percent better), and of those who improved, 27 percent were *really* improved (meaning 50-100 percent better). The *average* improvement, at 6 months, was found to be 48 percent.

This is the basic question that we were attempting to answer: *Is the presence of abnormal methylation chemistry important to the devel-*

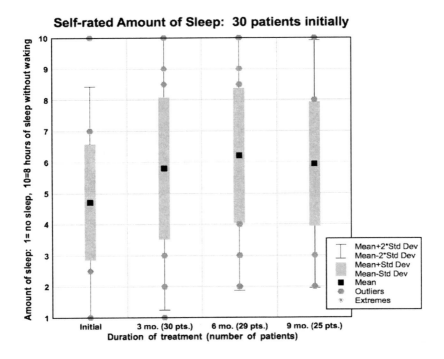

Figure 14.8   Improvement in Sleep with Methylation Protocol

opment of fibromyalgia and chronic fatigue? This has been answered with clarity: Yes. Clearly, abnormalities in methylation chemistry are common, almost universal, in our patients with chronic fatigue and fibromyalgia. And, here's the good news: they are also *treatable* with the use of a fairly simple group of supplements, taken once a day.

This was exciting new information, and we have just completed the next phase of this research. In the original project, all patients received exactly the *same* supplements for 6 months. But now, if we treat these patients separately and individually, based on their unique, measured biochemistry and genetic information, can they get even better?

To test this hypothesis, we continued treating the same patients

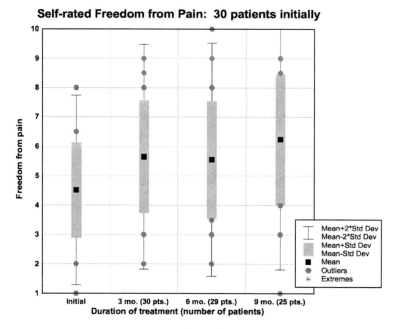

Figure 14.9 Decrease in Pain Rated as Freedom from Pain with
Methylation Protocol

we have just described, and with the expertise of Dr. Amy Yasko (who measured their genetic information), Dr. Rich van Konynenburg, and Dr. Tapan Audhya (the director of the Vitamin Diagnostics Laboratory), we formulated individual treatment programs unique to each patient. We based each treatment on the biochemical and genetic information that we had obtained from testing each patient, and we followed them for 3 additional months. We continued to test their chemistry and follow their clinical improvement with questionnaires.

What we discovered was that these patients *continued* to improve, particularly with the addition of Dr. Yasko's unique methylation treatment materials. We saw continued and significant rises in glutathione and SAM, and with it, patients had various degrees of clinical improvement. Several patients, who had only reported 10-15 percent initial improvement, now told us they were 50-60 percent better. One patient, who had not worked in over 5 years, was able to successfully resume full-time employment!

But that's not all. At the end of our program, based on research done by Sidney Baker, M.D., with autistic children, we added one more piece for 9 patients. Dr. Baker had discovered several years ago, that if he treated autistic children with elevated adenosine levels with Acyclovir (an anti-viral antibiotic with additional benefits to methylation chemistry), they improved. Well, 9 of our patients, who had gotten better, but not achieved optimal results, still had elevated adenosine levels at the end of 9 months of treatment. So I offered them an additional 2-3 months of a trial of the medication, Acyclovir, 200 mg, 5 times daily, and all of them agreed to try it. The results: 8 of the 9 patients reported an additional 20 percent improvement.

The upshot of all of this information is that these patients, who had experienced 30-60 percent improvement on our previous treatment program, were now describing 60-90 percent improvement on the completion of this study. From my perspective, there is no question that this represents a major new addition to our treatment options for these patients.

Now you can see why I'm so excited about methylation chemistry and why I am so eager for you to understand even a little of it. For example, you might read this material and realize how important it is to raise low glutathione levels. The obvious question would be "Why don't you just give these patients glutathione?" Well, that has been tried by numerous investigators, using glutathione in every form available: oral, intravenous, transdermal, even rectal. Although they have some benefit, these treatments don't hold and success is quite limited. It turns out that if the body is deficient in glutathione because it can't *make* it, giving it to the body in *any* form is merely a temporary fix (only hours, actually) and sends the body the wrong message. If the body *thinks* it has adequate glutathione, it stops making it, and that makes everything worse. So we have to restore the body's innate ability to *make* glutathione to achieve health. Our research results show that this is now possible.

I won't show you any more diagrams of how these cycles actually interact with other important cycles, most notably the ability to make the essential neurotransmitters serotonin and dopamine, which we explored in the previous chapter. An example of the importance of this chemistry is that our ability to make melatonin, essential for sleep, rests on our ability to *methylate* serotonin *into* melatonin. If this process is impaired, we can immediately see how sleep could be affected.

Although the chemistry we are discussing is complicated, the treatment is not. The use of this simplified methylation protocol, provided at the end of this chapter, has now been used by several physicians in hundreds of patients with excellent results, quite similar to mine. As this is a natural therapy, improvement is not immediate. While a few patients report some improvement within a few weeks, the average time it takes to begin to notice improvement is 6 weeks.

However, I must provide some words of warning. Although these natural materials have no known side effects, when they do work, they may dramatically improve the body's ability to process stored toxins. If that happens, toxins may be released into the system in amounts greater than the body's ability to deal with them, and these patients may initially get worse. Keep in mind that this is not a side effect; it reflects the fact that our treatment is working. These reactions are not rare. We have seen these reactions in up to 50 percent of our patients, varying from very mild (the usual reaction) to one that is quite severe. Usually, these reactions reflect an exacerbation of underlying symptoms, the most common being an increase in aches and pains and fatigue. A few have reported abdominal symptoms consisting of stomach cramping, constipation or diarrhea. A few have reported headache. These symptoms have usually resolved within a few days, once we have decreased the dosage or changed the frequency of administration from nightly to every other day, every third day, or in rare cases, once a week. Once the body adjusts to the lighter dosage, we can usually get our patients up to the full dosage and see the full benefits.

Please do not take this warning lightly. I truly believe that these supplements should only be taken under the direction of a knowledgeable, experienced medical professional with training in this area. As they say on television: "Please, folks, don't try this at home."

Edward's Story

This story not only describes benefits of methylation treatment, but in its complexity gives an excellent example of how these ideas come together to promote healing.

Edward was a medical student who came to see me in his last year of training. He had been "reasonably functional" until eighteen months prior, when he experienced the onset of waves of nausea, severe fatigue, difficulties with mental concentration and focus, and numbness and tingling around his mouth and left hand.

He had a complete evaluation by neurologists, gastroenterologists, and others. He did have adult-onset diabetes, which was carefully monitored. No real cause for his symptoms was uncovered by conventional testing, but Edward was obviously concerned, as these symptoms seriously impaired his ability to function as a medical student.

Edward had read about Wilson's Syndrome and found a local physician who started him on long-acting T3. On this, he began to feel somewhat better, especially with his memory and concentration, but his energy didn't really improve. Other relevant components of his history included a severe bout of mononucleosis in college with a recurrence several years later, documented sleep apnea, and a slip on the ice in his second year of medical school which injured his sacrum.

In response to measured low levels of DHEA and magnesium, bacterial pathogens in his GI tract, notably Klebsiella, and a visual contract (FACT) test which suggested neurotoxicity, we began treatment with DHEA, magnesium infusions, supplements for his bowel and digestion, transfer factors for the Epstein-Barr infection, and Welchol for presumed neurotoxicity. Osteopathic manipulation was also provided at each visit.

Edward improved somewhat on this regimen, but he still was so fatigued and mentally compromised that he was having difficulty completing his last few clinical rotations that would allow him to graduate from medical school. He was frightened that he would not be able to graduate and would not realize his dreams of becoming a physician. Since Edward was obviously a compassionate and bright young man, this would indeed have been tragic.

An unusually severe setback after a viral infection suggested that his immune system was compromised by adrenal deficiency, and testing for this revealed it to be true. We started him on Cortef, and he began to improve again. After four months, he was still not well enough to function adequately at school, so we began the methylation protocol along with the use of D-ribose for energy. Within two months, he was improved

enough that he successfully completed his studies and gradu-
ated from medical school. He was still not convinced that he
was well enough to begin his residency program (I shared
his concerns in that regard), so we measured his methylation
chemistry and, despite taking our supplement protocol for 3-4
months, he still had profoundly low glutathione and folic acid
levels (making us wonder how low it would have been had we
tested him before beginning the protocol).

When we added new supplements to improve his methyla-
tion chemistry, he got much better and was able to begin his
residency program as scheduled. He was very pleased that he
was able to work long hours, but was still just "getting by."
We measured his iodine levels and they were low, and when
we added Iodoral treatment, he had another obvious improve-
ment in his level of functioning. His tremors and numbness
and tingling sensations were virtually gone, and his visual
contrast (FACT) testing had returned to normal. At his last
visit, he remarked that he felt better than he had in years, de-
spite the long hours of work and training. He was able to go
to social functions and needed less sleep and naps. Although
not yet cured, he has been able to fully resume his life, and
we are confident that he will realize his dream of becoming a
complete physician.

Edward's story gives us a nice example of how we can take a step-
by-step approach to the treatment of these complex medical problems.
If we are patient and observant, we can figure out what we need to do
to restore these compromised patients back to health, and that, for me,
is truly fulfilling.

I would like to point out that we have tried this protocol with several patients who have reported to us that they have been depressed
since childhood, for no clear reason, and several have improved dramatically with its use. We have also used them with patients that have
autism, ADHD and ADD, with clinical benefits in most cases. Those
physicians who have been working with autism for some time (see

Chapter 22), are well aware of how important methylation chemistry is for those children.

You can see that we have just scratched the surface of the importance of methylation chemistry in health and illness and we are excited by the prospect of great strides in this new area of study.

Further Reading

Yasko, Amy, and Garry Gordon. *The Puzzle of Autism: Putting It All Together*. 2nd ed. Payson, AZ: Matrix, 2006.

METHYLATION PROTOCOL

Adapted from a treatment program developed by Amy Yasko, M.D., Ph.D.[1]

BASIC MATERIALS

1. Actifolate [2]: ¼ tablet (200mcg) daily
2. Intrinsi B12/folate [3]: ¼ tablet daily
3. General Vitamin Neurological Health Formula [4]: start with ¼ tablet and work up dosage as tolerated to 2 tablets daily
4. Phosphatidyl Serine Complex [5]: 1 softgel capsule daily
5. Activated B12 Guard [6]: 1 sublingual lozenge daily

PROTOCOL

The first two supplement tablets are difficult to break into quarters. We recommend that you obtain (from any pharmacy) a good-quality pill splitter to assist with this process. They can, alternatively, be crushed into powders, and then separated on a flat surface, and the powders can be mixed together. They can be taken orally with water, with or without food.

Occasionally these can make patients sleepy, so some take them at bedtime. They can be taken any time of day, with or without food.

Go slowly! Occasionally, as the methylation cycle blockages are released, toxins are released and processed by the body, and this can lead to an exacerbation of symptoms. If this happens, try smaller doses, every other day. Slowly work up to the full dosages.

[1] Yasko, Amy. *The Puzzle of Autism*. Bethel, ME: Neurological Research Institute, 2006.
[2] Actifolate is a registered trademark of Metagenics, Inc.
[3] Intrinsi B12/Folate is a registered trademark of Metagenics, Inc.
[4] General Vitamin Neurological Health Formula is formulated and supplied by Holistic Health Consultants LLC.
[5] Phosphatidyl Serine Complex, SerinAid, is a product of Olympian Labs.
[6] Activated B12 Guard is a registered trademark of Perque LLC.

❖ ❖ ❖

Pain

It would be a rare human being who had never experienced pain. Alas, it is an all-too-common part of our existence. For some fortunate individuals, pain is fleeting, minimal, and does not interfere with their day-to-day life. For others, pain becomes a life-long struggle and consumes them.

This section is devoted to an understanding of both acute and chronic pain. Like the rest of this book, it is not intended to present a comprehensive discussion of this subject; that could take volumes. Rather, it is my intent to describe the essentials of good pain diagnosis and treatment, and to single out a few specific treatments for discussion. To continue the theme of hope for those who have been told that nothing more can be done, I want to show how a different approach to diagnosis opens up whole new avenues of treatments that the reader may not have previously considered.

In our current medical system, part of the problem with evaluating pain is our emphasis on specialized care. Just last week I saw a young woman who had three different specialists for her neck pain, her mid-back pain, and her lower back pain! I can only describe this as fragmented care, and unless someone is looking at the bigger picture, the treatments of one physician may unwittingly be in conflict with those of another physician.

Each specialist naturally puts an emphasis on her own perspective (often to the exclusion of other considerations). So for the evaluation of low back pain, we would not be surprised to find the neurologist and neurosurgeon focusing on the nerves, or structures that impinge on nerves. And we would expect the orthopedist to focus on the bone structure and spurs. And we would expect the rheumatologist to focus on the joints. And we would expect the chiropractor to focus on body alignment and structure.

In my world, where patients with complicated problems turn up on my doorstep, pain is multi-factorial. That is to say, my patients' pains are produced by a complex interaction in the nerves, bones, joints, ligaments, tendons, and structural alignment, all of which interact with each other. Unless I can look at the whole picture, I, too, risk getting stuck in one area of perspective, and it is not likely that the problem can be accurately diagnosed or treated. Again, as throughout this book, diagnosis reigns supreme. My efforts, therefore, will go to looking at this pain problem from as many different perspectives as I can bring to the table.

We will begin this section with an overview of how to look at pain in this way, with an emphasis on how a whole body area needs to be evaluated and treated. I will then attempt to persuade you that a different model for treating acute pain is needed in an attempt to prevent recurrent or chronic pain. I would like to share with you a research study I completed five years ago in which we treated 250 consecutive cases of low back pain, and I hope this will clearly make my point.

Then, I would like to discuss two specific treatments with which you may not be familiar: osteopathic craniosacral manipulation and prolotherapy. This will hopefully give you some idea that other approaches do exist, and may be helpful in providing relief or cure for your pain problem.

Lastly, I would like to refer you to the Afterword section of this book, where some newer, cutting-edge treatments and therapies are briefly reviewed to give you even more ideas about what else may be possible.

❖ ❖ ❖

Chapter 15

Introductory Concepts for the Treatment of Pain

A Pain in the Derriere

*P*erhaps the most common complaint that patients express when they arrive in my office is that of pain. Low back pain, neck pain, shoulder pain, chest pain, abdominal pain, headache, and generalized pain (including fibromyalgia and arthritis) are of major concern for most of my patients, and the vast majority of them have already seen many other physicians and other healthcare providers for consultation before they arrive at my office. The very fact that these patients are in my office makes it clear that they have not had a satisfactory diagnosis or treatment, so obviously we must begin there.

It is my impression that since these patients have failed to improve with a wide variety of treatments, the single most frequent medical mistake in the treatment of pain is the lack of a clear diagnosis. Now this might seem obvious, but without a clear, concise understanding of the cause of a problem, how are we expected to formulate a viable treatment plan?

In the current language of pain specialists, when a patient presents with pain, we must search for the pain *generator*. Where, exactly, is this pain coming from? Let's take low back pain as an example, the commonest pain complaint seen by family physicians. When a patient points to her lower back and says, "It hurts right here," that should be just the beginning of our evaluation. Regrettably, in conventional medicine, with the limited amount of time available to evaluate any medical problem thoroughly, or even superficially, hasty diagnoses are made. This often pressures the time-challenged doctor to an off-the-cuff diagnosis of mechanical low back pain for this particular patient, which is far too vague to be of use in formulating a treatment plan. The conventional approach for this "disease," as we will discuss in our next chapter, is the prescription of pain medication or muscle relaxants. The patient then takes her prescription medications, and if she is lucky, the pain will go away on its own. These medications are not specific for the treatment of our patient; after all, we have not defined the specific tissues that have been injured here. Pain relievers and muscle relaxants only buy us a little time in which the tissues may heal on their own, if they are able to heal at all.

If the pain doesn't go away promptly, the next medical step is usually to provide physical therapy. Again, if the patient is lucky, he will be referred to a physical therapist who will take the time to look for the pain generator and specifically treat it. If the therapist finds the injured tissue—muscles, joints, ligaments, tendons, discs, nerves, or a combination of these—the treatment can be properly directed. Unfortunately, many physical therapists are under the same time pressures as physicians, and they usually apply non-specific remedies without a clear diagnosis, including ultrasound, neural stimulation, heat- or cold-based treatments, massage, and non-specific stretching exercises. Again, with this type of treatment program, a lucky patient will see the pain resolve on its own. But if not, the patient may then be referred to a physiatrist (a rehabilitation specialist), orthopedist, neurosurgeon, neurologist, anesthesiologist, or pain specialist, who may or may not attempt to make a specific diagnosis to begin definitive treatment.

Most of my patients tell me that although they have had x-rays, CT and MRI scans, nerve conduction tests, and have seen multiple specialists, no one has actually touched the affected area to examine it. While this may sound harsh, this has been reported to me so frequently over the past twenty years that I have come to believe my patients. This oversight in examination has been observed by many pain specialists and represents a major problem in the medical care that our pain patients receive. As obvious as it seems, one cannot make a clear diagnosis without actually touching or palpating the injured tissues to look for the pain generator. In our next chapter, we'll see that this problem has been compounded by the current medical belief that physicians *can't* make a clear diagnosis. So why should we even try?

Henry's Story

Henry was a prominent neurologist from Kansas who came to see me twelve years ago with what he described as low back pain. For the previous five years, he had seen an array of his colleagues, including orthopedists and neurosurgeons, who had diagnosed a bulging disc in his lower back as his pain's source. These specialists provided Henry with a variety of treatments. When his pain began five years before he came to me, an MRI scan showed the presence of a bulging disc, and he underwent surgery to remove the disc, with no relief of his pain or symptoms. Multiple steroid injections into the lower back had provided no relief. With the continuation of his pain, Henry became frustrated, and when a colleague mentioned to him that I might have a different approach, he came down for a visit.

When I asked Henry to describe his pain, he pointed to his right buttock and described a severe pain in that area, especially when he sat for too long. As he reflected on his symptoms, he recalled that this was actually his initial symptom, which really had not changed over this five-year period of time. This pain started in his right buttock and radiated down the back of his right leg to his calf, following the distribution of the sciatic nerve. When I examined him, he had no pain near or around the lower spine or sacroiliac joints. His pain could be reproduced by touching the right ischial tuberosity ("sitting bone"). The muscle directly above this region that spans the buttock, called the piriformis muscle, was in rather severe spasm.

This piriformis muscle is especially important when we evaluate patients who complain of sciatica, since the sciatic nerve often runs right through the body of this muscle. If that muscle tightens up or goes into spasm, it can pinch the sciatic nerve in a misguided effort to attempt to protect the nearby pain generator (in this case the ischial tuberosity, or sitting bone). In my experience, spasm of the piriformis muscle is by far the commonest cause of sciatica and is frequently overlooked as the source of sciatic symptoms; instead, most physicians focus their diagnostic efforts exclusively upon the lower lumbar spine. There is a bursa, or sac, which covers the ischial tuberosity to lubricate it and protect it from the friction of all the sitting we do. If that sac becomes inflamed, we call this an ischial tuberosity bursitis, which is just a fancy term for bursitis of the sitting bones.

I told Henry that I thought this was his diagnosis and that it could explain all of his symptoms. I offered him a simple injection of cortisone into the ischial tuberosity region, along with an injection of Marcaine, a long-acting local anesthetic, into the irritated trigger points of the piriformis muscle, which Henry accepted. We then followed these injections with a stretching of that muscle so that it could resume its normal resting length.

Having spent the past five years wrestling with this pain and looking exclusively at the lower spine as its cause, Henry was a bit skeptical that this would work. No one had ever proposed this diagnosis to him, and no one had ever examined his buttock before, either. I performed this simple procedure with his full co-operation (which took all of three minutes), and for the first time in five years George reported immediate and complete relief of his pain. Still shaking his head and doubting that this would last, he discovered that this relief actually lasted for several weeks. He returned three weeks after his first visit for a second injection; after that, the pain disappeared completely, and it never returned. Henry was a happy camper. He subsequently referred quite a few patients to my office for evaluation and treatment of their pain.

Henry's story emphasizes some of the points I have been trying to make. Despite the fact that Henry was a specialist and well aware of the various possible causes of lower back pain, he was so caught up in the conventional medical model that it somehow never occurred to him that he and his treating colleagues were on the wrong track. Even surgery had proven ineffective. The real problem was that no one had actually examined his area of pain. Once the pain generators had been identified, specific treatment could be provided, allowing healing to occur. Henry spent five years in pain and underwent unnecessary surgery because this basic principle of medicine was not followed.

Our bodies are complicated, but if we study them, they usually make a great deal of sense. It is a cliché to say that everything is connected to everything else, but if we forget this simple fact, we are missing out on the full medical picture. The lower back, which we've been discussing, is an excellent example of this. Figure 15.1 below illustrates the main players that affect this region.

The most common pain generator in the lower back, from my experience, is an injury to the sacroiliac joint. Patients with these injuries usually complain of pain right over that joint. They may also complain of pain radiating down their leg, or over the lower back muscles, or of the lower rib cage on that side, or of a deep pain in their groin. How do

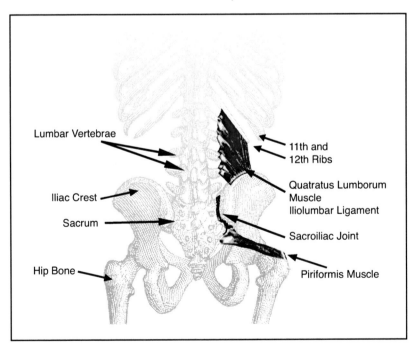

Figure 15.1   Illustration of the Lower Back Region

we explain all of that? It's actually quite simple: we must understand the anatomical connections.

In Figure 15.1, you can see that there are several ways in which the body may try to manage sacroiliac joint pain: it may tighten up the piriformis muscle, as we discussed above, which may pinch the sciatic nerve and cause pain to radiate down that leg. The piriformis muscle is paired with the psoas muscle that spans the groin. If the piriformis muscle contracts or goes into spasm, so will the psoas muscle, which will cause pain in the groin area. Additionally, the muscle above the sacroiliac joint, the quadratus lumborum (the thick lower back muscle which most people think of as their main back muscle) may tighten up, with the same protective reflex. The quadratus lumborum, in turn, is attached to the lower rib cage just above it. Yanking tight on those ribs, the quadratus lumborum may pull on the ribs with enough force that it can jam the joints with which those ribs attach to the spine, and this sets off rib cage pain.

Treatment of this common form of lower back pain is based on an understanding of these muscles' interactions. The patients' descriptions of their pain areas lead us quickly to understand which part(s) of this system we need to focus on. If pain is radiating down the leg, we need to look at the piriformis muscle. If the pain is in the groin area in front, we need to examine the psoas muscle. If the pain is described in the lower rib cage area, we need to examine the quadratus lumborum muscle and the lower ribs. Often we need to examine all of these areas to clarify how they are interacting. Here's the important part: once we have identified which tissues are producing our patient's pain, *we need to treat them all*. That is, we cannot just inject the sacroiliac joint if that is the main cause of pain, but we must also treat the jammed ribs and all of the associated muscles that are in spasm. Then the whole system can settle down and heal.

If we miss just one component of the problem, it may aggravate the lower back, and although the patient may initially improve, her symptoms will keep coming back. Our patients are often the perfect guides to what we may have missed; if we are really listening to them, they will tell us that some of their symptoms have improved, but they are left with different symptoms now. That description will point us to the next area that requires treatment.

I call this process *layering*. What hurts the patient most will get all of his attention. It's sort of like the old adage, "The wheel that squeaks gets the grease." There may be other painful areas, but the worst may be the only one that grabs the patient's awareness. If we remove that pain, often we find another pain below that. Sometimes patients get frustrated by this and tell me the pain has moved. Usually it hasn't actually *moved*. We are merely becoming aware of the next layer, and this can get our full attention for healing. It usually doesn't take more than a few layer removals to provide substantial healing.

Now that you are aware of these basic principles, let us take a more detailed look at our treatment options.

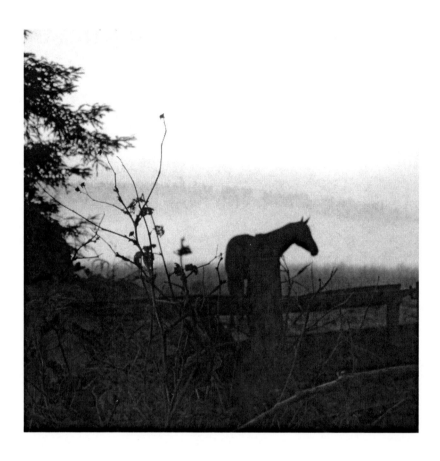

Chapter 16

Can Chronic Pain Be Prevented?

An Ounce of Prevention . . .

There exists in the current practice of medicine an odd prevailing misconception: not only does acute pain *not* need to be treated aggressively, but the cause of acute pain cannot be accurately diagnosed; hence, even designing a treatment is futile. Some of you may think this is an exaggeration, but I can promise you it's not.

R.A. Deyo has written extensively on this problem of diagnosis and treatment of pain. He asserts that "up to 85% of patients with low back pain cannot be given a definitive diagnosis because of the poor association among symptoms, pathological findings, and imaging results." The current accepted model for treatment of acute low back pain was developed by the Agency for Healthcare Research and Quality (AHRQ). This consensus organization has reviewed the available research in this field and has concluded that the initial assessment of patients with acute low back pain should focus on the detection of "red flags." These flags are time-honored findings and symptoms that suggest serious or life-threatening causes and include conditions in which spinal nerves are pinched or damaged. Red flags, according to the AHRQ, include bulging discs that impinge upon the nerves or spinal cord, metatstatic cancers, or spinal stenosis. If these are not diagnosed and treated promptly, we would all agree that our patients would be subject to significant harm. Red flags can also include the loss of bowel or bladder control, loss of sensation or strength in one or both extremities, or loss of reflexes. Medical practitioners, myself included, agree completely with the need for looking for and treating these red flags. However, when we understand that only 2 to 3 percent of patients show these particular symptoms, we realize that the vast majority of patients with back injury, without red flags, will not receive that kind of attention.

In the absence of these red flags, the AHRQ has proposed that imaging studies and further testing of patients with acute low back pain are not usually helpful in the first four weeks following injury. They suggest that relief of discomfort can be accomplished most safely with nonprescription medication and/or spinal manipulation. Bed rest for more than four days is not recommended, and patients are encouraged to return to work or their normal daily activities as soon as possible. What this means is that if you are suffering from acute low back pain and you don't have one of these red flags, your doctor will probably tell you to take some ibuprofen or Tylenol and get back to work as soon as possible.

Having worked with the treatment of pain for many years, both acute and chronic, I felt this concept made little sense. More important, it did not fit with my own observations that a precise diagnosis of acute pain was entirely possible and essential to correct treatment. With exact, early, aggressive treatment, it was my impression that patients did quite well, and it was rare to see the onset of chronic pain afterward. Conventional medical wisdom says, "Statistics reveal that approximately 10 percent of patients with back pain complaints do not get better in 4 to 6 weeks," and "more than half the people who recover from a first episode of acute low back pain will have another episode within a few years. Their problems with back pain become chronic."

So in 1999, in order to delve deeper into this subject, I embarked on a research project. This entailed taking a part-time position with a clinic specializing in occupational medicine, a clinic that contracted with the largest employers in our area. What made this particularly relevant was that we were working with a captive audience: in these large companies, all of the injuries and pains sustained on the job had to be reported to the employer, and they had to come to us for evaluation and treatment. This gave us excellent access to follow-up care. I was assigned to evaluate only those severely injured patients who had suffered acute pain injuries and were not responding to our routine care. So, we evaluated and treated 250 consecutive patients with acute low back pain and another 100 consecutive patients with acute injuries to their neck, thoracic spine, and head areas. We kept careful records of our treatment results, including return-to-work data and whether these same patients came back to our clinic with recurrent symptoms within a three-year period. As we discuss the concepts of pain in this chapter, I will often refer to my experiences at this clinic.

Before I relate the results of that four-year study, let's start with understanding, if we can, why conventional medicine does not believe in an accurate preliminary diagnosis. You may not like the answer, but it's simple: most physicians are not trained to examine the musculoskeletal system with their hands, so they overly rely on x-rays, CTs, and MRIs to make their diagnosis. Unfortunately, in this regard, these testing methods are a little crude. MRIs, for example, are unable to distinguish small but significant structural abnormalities of 2 mm or less. So for larger structural problems, like a protruding disc, they are excellent, but to detect a muscle that is in spasm or a slight spinal or joint abnormality, MRIs simply don't have the visual resolution to make the diagnosis. But our hands do.

Although I'm an M.D., I've been blessed with some wonderful osteopathic and chiropractic teachers who have taken the time to teach me how to feel for and treat these problems. With this information and hands-on treatment, we can make presumptive diagnoses about exactly where our patients' pain is coming from. We can then get clear feedback from their response to our treatment, which will further clarify whether our diagnosis is correct or not.

Here is a simple example. As mentioned in our last chapter, the most common acute injury in my experience is that of acute sacroiliac joint strain. First of all, the injured patient will point to those joints when she describes her pain, and when I examine her, I find that those areas are much more tender than the surrounding tissues. I can then inject the sacroiliac joints with a mixture of Marcaine (a long acting anesthetic) and cortisone (for longer relief of inflammation), and I find that if the diagnosis is correct, the patient reports immediate decrease in pain. Over several days, this pain decreases or disappears completely. To me, this is pretty good presumptive evidence that we did identify the source of pain and treat it correctly. In this way, we can systematically go over the entire area of pain and come up with a clear diagnosis.

How the patient responds to the treatment makes it quite clear how accurate the diagnosis actually was.

Keep in mind that in an injured patient, it is not always that simple. The injured tissues are connected to other tissues, which may also be injured. We have to look at the whole picture. For example, in a patient with an injured sacroiliac joint on one side, the muscles that surround the injured tissue usually tighten or go into spasm as the body attempts to protect the injured area. As we discussed in our previous chapter, in this case, the quadratus lumborum (the thick muscles on the sides of the lower back) tighten, pull on the lower ribs, and often jam them. All of this leads to pain in the lower rib cage area. The piriformis muscle across the buttock and its companion muscle, the psoas (in the front of the groin), also tighten to protect the area, and the pain may radiate into those areas as well. Commonly, the sciatic nerve runs through the piriformis muscle, and when that muscle contracts protectively, it literally *pinches* the sciatic nerve, causing pain to radiate down the patient's leg. So, we have to take all this into account and treat it all: not just the sacroiliac joint. Figure 16.1 shows a posterior (back) view of this area and illustrates this relationship.

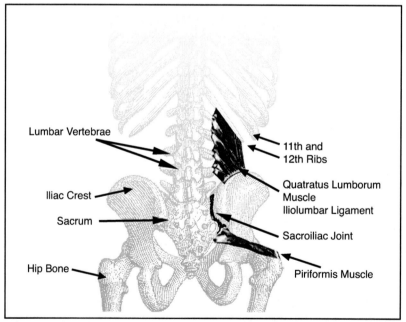

Figure 16.1   The Anatomy of the Quadratus and Periformis Muscles

Take, for example, a badly injured worker with severe right-sided sacroiliac pain. He also experiences accompanying spasms of the piriformis, psoas, and quadratus lumborum muscles, as well as jammed ribs of the right lower rib cage. He will therefore present to us complaining of pain that is worse in the right sacroiliac joint area, but also radiates up into the right lower rib cage, down the right leg, and into the right groin. A comprehensive approach to treating this problem would include—

- An injection of the upper and lower poles of the right sacroiliac joint
- Osteopathic manipulation of the sacroiliac joint, especially if ilial rotation (a hip that is out of alignment) is present
- Release of the jammed ribs on the right side
- A muscular release of the spasm in the piriformis, quadratus lumborum, and psoas tissues
- Trigger-point injections or myofascial release techniques that perhaps would require the identification of and treatment of other affected muscle groups, such as the gluteus muscles or tensor fascia lata

You can see that this would be a far cry from simply offering ibuprofen for four weeks and waiting to see if it worked or not. The exact treatment, of course, would depend on the exact tissues that were found to be injured by our careful evaluation. If my patient responds well to the specific treatments I provide to those areas, it is a pretty safe bet that those were indeed the injured tissues. This makes me quite certain that a specific tissue diagnosis for low back injuries is entirely possible, and, in fact, *necessary* for correct treatment.

That was precisely our approach at the occupational medicine clinic that I joined in 1999. Each patient was carefully evaluated and then treated by myself and a team of others, which included another physician trained in osteopathic manipulation. Each injured area was treated with methods suited to the nature of that injury: injections, osteopathic manipulation, medication, physical therapy, and combinations of those modalities.

Sources of Pain in 243 Consecutive Patients	
Sacroiliac Joint	80%
Piriformis Muscle	21%
Quadratus Muscle	20%
Rib Head Pain	10%
Other Muscles (Psoas, Gluteus)	
Ligament Injury	6%
Somatic Dysfunction	4%
Herniated Disc	3.2%
Facet Joint	3%
Ilial Rotation	3%
Ischial Tuberosity Bursitis	2%
Greater Trochanteric Bursitis	2%
Sacrococcygeal Injury	2%
Iliolumbar Ligament	1.5%
Chronic Low Back Pain (Non Specific)	1%
Spinal Stenosis	0.5%

Table 16.1   Pain Generators for Acute Low Back Pain

What did we learn through using these methods? Table 16.1 above shows the discoveries we made about the nature of pain generators.

If you total the percentages in this table, it is clear that this is greater that 100 percent. This is because, as I have been stressing, each patient often has more than one pain generator. You can see that injury to the sacroiliac joint was by far the most common injury component, and that a herniated disc, which is what most patients fear most, was present only 3.2 percent of the time. This percentage is compatible with most studies in the medical literature.

More important, we found that of our recently injured low back patients, only 18 of 243 came back to the clinic with a recurrence of back pain over a three-year follow up. This represents a re-injury rate of only 7.3 percent, whereas national statistics suggest that in patients treated by the conventional, non-aggressive medical model, the re-injury rate was closer to 50 percent! This is quite significant, so much that it suggests that our aggressive approach to treating acute pain prevented most relapses.

We followed our patients for at least three years after their original injury, and only eight of them (3.7 percent) went on to develop chronic pain, whereas by national statistics, this should have been much higher. To be more specific, "statistics reveal that approximately 10% of patients with back pain complaints do not get better in 4-6 weeks" and that "more than half the people who recover from a first episode of acute low back pain will have another episode within a few years. Their problems with back pain become chronic" [1]. You can see that we clearly demonstrated a marked reduction in both recurrence of pain and the onset of chronic pain.

We also followed another 100 consecutive patients with other injury-related pains, including spinal injuries involving the cervical or neck area, thoracic or mid-back area, and injuries to the head. As you can see from Tables 16.2 and 16.3, our results imply that most common bodily injuries respond well to this treatment process and also suggest that the diagnosis-based aggressive treatment approach that I am advocating may not only improve the rapidity of healing, but also may prevent recurrent or chronic pain in most cases.

Consecutive Acutely Injured Patients (N=364)		
BODY AREA	REINJURY	CHRONIC
Lower Back 243 patients	18 (7.4%)	8 (3.2%)
Neck/Shoulder 71 patients	1	2
Thoracic/Ribs 39 patients	6	1
Head 11 patients	0	1
Total: 364 Patients	25 (6.9%)	12 (3.3%)

Table 16.2   Consecutive Acutely Injured Patients

Acute Low Back Pain Aggressive Treatment 243 Consecutive Patients		
Reinjury	18 patients	7.4%
Chronic Pain	8 patients	3.2%

Table 16.3   Acute Low Back Pain Aggressive Treatment

We also looked at how quickly our patients went back to work. Since we were working in an occupational medicine clinic, this was of great interest to the employers who paid us for our work. Table 16.4 below shows our findings.

Spinal Injuries Return-to-Work Status		
	Return to Modi-fied Work	Return to Regular Work
Low Back Pain (n=243)	3.8 days	24.2 days
All Pain (n=364)	3.5 days	23.5 days

Table 16.4 Time from Onset of Injury to Resumption of Part-time and Full-time Work

Unfortunately, there are very few good statistics available that would allow us to compare our results with those of others who have treated injured workers with acute low back pain by different strategies. Although we don't have those numbers, I can say from my long years of work in this field that the return to modified work in an average of 3.8 days ("light duty") and the eventual resumption of regular work in an average of 24.2 days ("regular duty") was impressive to the employers with whom we worked. They became quite pleased with our results. Keep in mind that in this study we only treated the more seriously injured patients, making these numbers look even better.

The costs of chronic pain are well documented in terms of personal and familial losses, with staggering financial losses for both the individual and society. Our study suggests that this new model of understanding acute pain may lead to a whole different approach to treatment, which, in most cases, may prevent the pain from recurring or becoming chronic. Now doesn't that sound a lot better than taking a patient with acute pain, giving her ibuprofen for four weeks, and just hoping she'll get better?

Further Reading

Ashburn, Michael A., and Linda J. Rice, eds. *The Management of Pain*. New York: Churchill Livingstone, 1998.

Deyo, R A. "Fads in the Treatment of Low Back Pain." *The New England Journal of Medicine* 325.14 (1991): 1039–40.

Spilzer, Walter O. *Scientific Approach to the Assessment and Management of Activity-related Spinal Disorders*. Philadelphia: Harper & Row, 1987.

[1] Bigos, S., et al. *Acute Low Back Problems in Adults*. Clinical Practice Guidelines, Quick Reference Guide No. 14, AHCPR pub. 95-0643. U.S. Department of Health and Human Services, Public Health Service. Rockville, MD: Agency for Health Care Policy and Research, 1994.

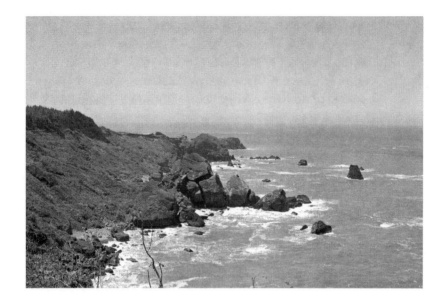

Chapter 17

Osteopathic Manipulation and Craniosacral Therapy

Lend Me a Hand

*L*et us explore the role of touch in healing. From my perspective, the act of making physical contact with another human being allows us to convey something that words cannot. Our touch, well beyond words, may speak volumes about our concerns for and feelings about our patients. I find that many of my patients arrive in our office somewhat jaded, having experienced bad medical visits for quite some time. They have spent a great deal of time and money looking for a cure, yet often they feel unheard, even hopeless. Many of their physicians have suggested, "There is nothing wrong with you," implying that their problems are essentially psychological.

While trying to stay hopeful, many patients are probably expecting more of the same from me, too. They have heard lots of words, lots of jargon, and lots of verbiage. Surprisingly, despite hours and hours of office visits, most patients have rarely or never been touched or carefully examined by their doctors. So if my patient experiences pain in a particular area, I will make every effort not only to examine that area thoroughly at the first visit, but to begin the process of treating it with manipulation. I have found that being touched by someone who genuinely cares, especially when it leads to immediate (even if temporary) improvement, conveys more than all of my words ever could. The act of physical contact carries the possibility of breaking through communication barriers and establishing a relationship on a deeper level. This is an excellent way to begin a therapeutic alliance, and, alas, one often neglected by my profession.

Manual medicine has been around for thousands of years, and it exists in a bewildering variety of forms or styles. But it is not my intention to catalogue these in any detail here; rather, I will simply provide an overview of this field to give the reader a sense of what can be achieved when the healing capacities of human touch are harnessed. Manual medicine is defined separately by each therapeutic discipline that provides it. Hence, there are osteopathic, chiropractic, physical therapy, massage, Ayurvedic, Rolfing, myotherapy, Shiatsu, and countless other forms of treatment. As the name *manual medicine* implies, practitioners use part(s) of their body to change specific musculoskeletal imbalances in the patient. Practitioners typically use their hands, but elbows, feet, and other body parts can also be utilized. The basic idea is that structural problems in the patient can be influenced and treated by either directly or indirectly working upon them. By structure, I simply mean imbalances and dysfunctions of specific anatomical areas: muscles, tendons, ligaments, bones, joints, connective tissues, and nerves.

Let's say you wake up in the morning and you've somehow slept "wrong" on your pillow. Now you've got a "crick" in your neck—it doesn't turn or rotate normally, and it hurts. As the morning moves along, you notice not only pain in the neck area, with restricted motion of your neck, but a headache starts up and your shoulders begin to ache and become tense. What should you do? If you sought conventional medical attention, you might be told you have a muscle spasm, which would be the correct medical diagnosis, and you'd probably be given pain medication or a muscle relaxant to take. After several days, your pain would probably go away slowly. But if you were aware of the benefits of manual medicine and sought out that form of treatment, you would find a more specific and speedier form of relief.

My first introduction to manipulation came early in my career when I had the privilege of working with Stan Weisenberg, a wonderful chiropractor, who shared my office space. While I noticed that my medication-treated patients took seven to ten days to get better, Stan's patients were getting better within a day or two, following his manipulative treatment of their necks and shoulders. So I begged him to teach me how to do it. Although we were friends, the climate of distrust between physicians and chiropractors in the early 1970s was such that Stan later confessed to me that he had to get up some courage to teach me; he was concerned that I might somehow view his work negatively. The opposite was true. I was astonished to observe how he could restore patients back to health with carefully orchestrated treatment, and I began to learn how to manipulate necks and lower backs. It soon became obvious that my patients were now getting better much more quickly, and I started studying other types of manipulative medicine as well.

Stan and I had a mutual teacher of Reichian therapy (not to be confused with Reiki, which is a form of energy treatment) who encouraged me to study osteopathic craniosacral manipulation. This was a branch of osteopathy to which they, as chiropractors, did not have access as it was taught only to osteopaths, M.D. physicians, and dentists.

So, in 1975, I went to Colorado Springs to spend a very intense week with a roomful of superb healers, who kindly and gently began the process of instructing me. It is hard to convey how presumptuous my presence in that class was at the time: I had very, very little manipulative training and knowledge; in fact, I didn't even know what an osteopath was. I had no idea that they were physicians trained just as rigorously as I had been, but that they had also studied the art of manipulation in the service of healing. What I did recognize at that first course was that these physicians were really good at what they did. I saw them do things with their hands that I had never dreamt possible. They opened up doors that completely changed my life.

The most fascinating concept of that initial experience was to learn that the cranial bones were not fused together throughout life, as my medical teaching had suggested, but that these bones were designed from birth to move and to literally "breathe." Of course, this motion is exquisitely minute, but I was taught how to perceive it and work with it to restore normal motion in the bones, which translated into improved motion of the tissues to which the bones are attached.

When I left Colorado Springs, I was unsure of how useful this information would be, or how well I could apply it. A week after my return to practice, I would see a patient who would clarify it for me. I was working in the emergency room of our local hospital, and a young boy came in who had been playing shortstop in a Little League game. A ball had been hit to him and took a bad hop, striking him sharply in the left jaw. He immediately noticed loss of hearing from his right ear and severe pain, tingling, and numbness of his right jaw. Had I not taken this course in craniosacral manipulation, I would have assumed some vague mechanism of injury and told the family to go home and be patient, hoping that his injury would somehow wear off by itself, over time. Instead, with my newfound knowledge, I could clearly see how the force of the injury to his left jaw had been transmitted into his right temporomandibular (jaw) joint and "jammed" his temporal bone, affecting his ear and causing all of his symptoms.

Using craniosacral therapy, I simply freed up his right temporal bone and jaw joint. My treatment consisted of inserting one gloved finger into the boy's mouth, while I held onto his cheekbone on the same side with my other hand. Inside his mouth, I applied a tiny amount of upward traction on his sphenoid bone, which I accessed by resting my little finger behind his upper teeth, while I rotated his cheek bone away from its "jammed" position. I then changed the position of my intraoral fingers to grasp his right lower jaw, and I applied gentle traction downward, freeing up his jaw joint. Within seconds, all of his symptoms disappeared. I was amazed. More important, I realized how useful this information was going to be and launched into an even deeper study and appreciation of this whole field.

Since my own study of manual medicine has been primarily osteopathic, I'd like to focus on the principles of this form of treatment. The first principle of osteopathic treatment as enunciated by founder A.T. Still in the late 1800s is, "The rule of the artery is supreme." Initially, this might sound a little vague, or obscure, but let's explore it a bit more. Dr. Still was referring to the fact that anything that compresses or restricts arterial blood flow in

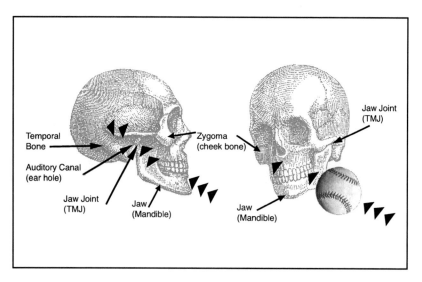

Figure 17.1   Diagram illustrating the mechanism of injury

any way prevents oxygen from reaching the tissues supplied by the arteries. These tissues would include muscles, tendons, ligaments, bones, nerves, and organs. In essence, every tissue must receive free, unrestricted arterial blood flow for optimal functioning. By identifying with precision all areas of restriction, a trained osteopath can restore blood flow to those tissues and powerfully influence the restoration of health. Dr. Still was referring to more than just arteries, however. His rule actually applies to all areas of flow within the body. Anything that restricts those flows—whether that flow is arterial, veinous, lymphatic, neuronal, respiratory, or even energetic—needs to be identified and freed up. The free, unrestricted flow of all fluids in the body is thus one important and often overlooked aspect of health. We can expand that concept to include the ability of the body to freely expand and contract and move (which even includes free flow on a cellular or biochemical level) as one direction in which we wish to move toward health. This rule of "the artery is supreme" is indeed a profound concept, and when applied toward healing, it is well worthy of prolonged study.

Identifying these restrictions, then, becomes a most important part of the healing process and is an essential feature of osteopathic treatment. Once again, we are talking about clear diagnosis, which can lead to a very specific, precise treatment plan. Whether we find a tight muscle, fascial strain (the fascia is the connective tissue that surrounds the muscles), bone or joint restricted in its motion, or a nerve that is impinged upon by other structures, we can find multiple methods of relieving these using the wide variety of manipulative techniques available to us.

I believe this is an underutilized component of healing. While conventional medicine barely recognizes the existence of this branch of healing, patients for centuries have been aware that physical touch can relieve pain, and they have sought those with skills in this area for comfort and healing and have often received the help they were looking for.

Heidi's Story

Heidi was a thirty-seven-year-old woman who had been suffering with constant daily pain located over her right cheek area and across the bridge of her nose, involving the front of her face below her nose and her upper and lower teeth. This had progressed over a seven-year period to include frequent headaches across her temples.

By the time I saw her, Heidi had already seen many excellent neurologists, neurosurgeons, and several other physicians who had prescribed every medication under the sun. None of the medications really helped, and many of them caused her significant side effects. She had received a steroid injection to a branch of the right maxillary nerve, under her right cheek, about a year previously. That area was still numb and tingling, as the injection had not relieved any of her pain like both she and her physician had hoped. She also described persistent pain in her low back and sacral areas. As we explored the cause of these symptoms in detail, Heidi really didn't know what had set it off those many years ago. The pain had become debilitating, and the constant wrestling with it had left her exhausted, making it difficult for her to take care of her children and husband and function well in her career as a therapist.

When I evaluated Heidi from a craniosacral perspective, she had marked restriction of motion of her whole cranial mechanism, especially the facial bones and a significant restriction of motion of her sacrum as well. (There is a direct anatomical connection between the sacrum and the base of the skull so that these are very closely related; restriction of one can easily affect the other.) Treatments involved freeing up her neck and shoulders and upper ribs (tightness in those areas affects the cranial structures) and extensive work with the cranial and facial bones. This included gentle traction upon all of the cranial bones, along with work inside her mouth to free up the cheek, sinus, and jaw restrictions, as well as work upon her sacrum and lower back tissues. As I treated her osteopathically every two weeks in all these areas, she slowly improved. Within four months of treatment, she reported to me that she was 85 percent better. She would go whole days where she experienced almost no pain at all. She also experienced improved energy and sleep and marked relief from her back pain. After a few more months of osteopathic treatments, she described 95 percent improvement.

Interestingly, after our first few treatments Heidi recalled having injured herself on two occasions from falls she had incurred. In one fall she struck her right cheekbone, and in the other she had fallen directly upon her face, particularly affecting both her upper and lower teeth. These areas that she injured were exactly the areas that were now causing her so much pain. The process of freeing up injured tissues often releases the memory of how the injury occurred. It is fascinating to observe how frequently we find this to occur when we treat with manual medicine. Patients are often surprised that they have somehow forgotten important parts of their history that help to explain their symptoms. We refer to this phenomenon as tissue memory, which reflects the fact that the memories are actually contained in the injured tissues, and not simply in the mind, as most people believe. Furthermore, emotions that may be connected to this injury are often bound up in the myofascial tissues themselves. The process of treating those injured tissues often brings forth the emotions that have been held in those tissues so that they can be expressed. This emotional release often greatly contributes to the healing process.

I believe that Heidi would not have recovered without this form of treatment. Time alone (seven years' worth in this case) did not cure. Precise identification of the cause(s) of her pain was essential to her healing. With the benefit of that precise diagnosis, we had the tools we needed to be of service.

Nothing is as simple as it sounds, unfortunately. For those of you who are thinking of seeking a qualified practitioner of craniosacral therapy, please be aware that there are several schools that teach this procedure and that there are significant differences between these schools. The original information on this subject was discovered and thoroughly researched by William Garner Sutherland, D.O., who single-handedly put this curriculum together over many decades. Therefore, the osteopathic craniosacral teachings have the longest history and usage, and are the most detailed and sophisticated, but have only been taught to D.O.s, M.D.s, and dentists. An osteopathic physician named John Upledger simplified this teaching and has made it available to chiropractors, physical therapists, massage therapists, and lay healers. By its basic nature, it can help with simple structural problems, but any complicated or sensitive structural problems may require the services of the full osteopathic training program for healing. In fact, if applied incorrectly, or in a heavy-handed fashion by those not properly trained, one can actually jam the sutures and do harm to the membrane and fluid physiology, injuring or damaging the patient. So be sure to delve into the training background of an individual who claims to do this form of therapy. It may sound like a bit of a cliché, but all craniosacral practitioners are not created equal, and that principle can be expanded to include virtually any treatment technique that you might seek. No practitioner should be offended by your inquiries into their training background; that information should be offered freely and comfortably.

In virtually every pain problem, we see a structural component. Many practitioners of medicine focus on the emotional components of pain, unfortunately conveying to the patient that they believe the problem is in the patient's head. Far too often, a careful evaluation of the long-injured tissues, which include muscles, fascia, joints, bones, and nerves, has not been performed. So if you have a long-standing pain problem, this is an area that you may well wish to explore.

Further Reading

Copland-Griffiths, Michael. *Dynamic Chiropractic Today: The Complete and Authoritative Guide to This Major Therapy.* San Francisco: HarperCollins, 1991.

Magoun, Harold. *Osteopathy in the Cranial Field.* Kirksville, MO: Journal Printing, 1966.

Prudden, Bonnie. *Pain Erasure.* New York: Ballantine, 1980.

Rolf, Ida. *Rolfing: The Integration of Human Structures.* New York: Harper & Row, 1977.

Travell, Janet, and David Simons. *Myofascial Pain and Dysfunction: The Trigger Point Manual.* Baltimore, MA: Williams and Wilkins, 1983. *(This superb two-volume book describes in wonderful detail the ways in which pain can radiate in a wide variety of patterns from a specific muscle group, and how to treat it. I've often said that if I were stranded on an island and had only a few medical textbooks at my disposal, this would be one of them.)*

Upledger, John E., and Jon Vredevoogd. *Craniosacral Therapy.* Seattle, WA: Eastland, 1983.

To find a practitioner of craniosacral manipulation in your area, visit The Cranial Academy's website at www.cranialacademy.com, or call (317) 594-0411 for a referral.

❖ ❖ ❖

Chapter 18

Prolotherapy

No Pain, No Gain

*I*n addition to craniosacral therapy and other forms of manual medicine, there is another highly underutilized treatment for chronic pain conditions: *prolotherapy*. This treatment technique has been around since the 1940s, when it was called *sclerotherapy*, but it has recently increased in popularity. It consists of a series of injections into ligaments or tendon insertions, which are designed to make these tissues stronger and tighter. The name *prolo* is a shortened form of the word *proliferate*, a clear description of what is occurring on a cellular and tissue level.

In prolotherapy, a mildly irritating solution is injected into the ligaments or tendons of the body, and at the site of that injection, we intentionally irritate and inflame those tissues. This in turn stimulates the natural healing forces of the body to bring new cells, called *fibroblasts*, into the inflamed tissues to deal with this inflammatory process. The fibroblasts grow, or *proliferate*, in the ligaments we have injected. The growth of these fibroblasts creates a thicker, stronger ligament or tendinous insertion, which, as we shall soon see, directly promotes healing. Studies have been done in rabbits showing that ligaments can potentially grow 40 percent stronger by using this treatment. Humans respond beautifully to this method, and it is the only method I know of in which a ligament can truly be strengthened. Muscles, of course, can be strengthened by a wide variety of exercises. But ligaments, as they are an entirely different type of tissue, do not respond to the kinds of treatments so useful for muscles. The good news is that we now have, through prolotherapy, a way to heal damaged ligaments.

You may not be aware of how essential ligaments are in all joint functioning. The integrity of every joint in the body is created by and composed of ligaments. When a ligament becomes stretched or damaged, it is no longer capable of holding the joint together properly. Frictional forces start to wear away the smooth cartilage surfaces that cover the opposing bones that create the joint. Thus, the process of arthritis begins. When this erosion of cartilage becomes severe, we call it *bone-on-bone,* meaning that the cartilage has worn away so completely that the bones are now rubbing against each other. In a normal joint, the bones and the cartilage that covers them are held apart by the tight ligaments, allowing the lubricating fluid in the joint space to keep these tissues healthy.

Let's take a look at the knee joint, depicted in Figure 18.1, as a good description of this process. On the left, we see a normal joint with tight ligaments that hold the joint spaces apart. Since we usually associate tightness with pain and strain, it's important to appreciate that this is the normal tension in the ligament and is essential to its functioning. If the ligaments become weak, as in the drawing on the right, the joint space collapses and the bones start to rub against each other, eventually creating an arthritic condition.

If we can stimulate these weakened ligaments to tighten, we can literally start to pull the bones that have collapsed into the joint space apart, thereby recreating the normal joint space and normalizing the joint function. As long as the damage has not gone on for too long, we have the wonderful possibility of treating arthritis of any joint in a preventive manner, by using prolotherapy. It allows us to put off, sometimes indefinitely, the need for surgery or joint replacement, and it markedly cures or reduces the joint pain we call arthritis.

Virtually any joint can be treated with prolotherapy. Let's take, for example, one of the most commonly injured joints: the sacroiliac joint. This joint is located in the lower back area between the sacrum (the thick triangle of bone at the base of the spine) and the two hip

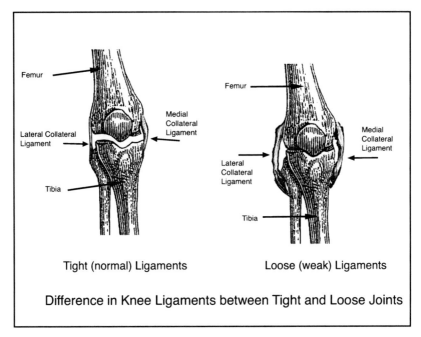

Figure 18.1 Structure of the Knee Joint

bones, which are medically referred to as the *ilia*, hence the technical term *sacroiliac*. Often patients refer to this area as their hips, but technically that is not correct; the hip refers to the joint between the femur (the lower leg bone) and the acetabulum (the area in the pelvis to which it attaches). Lower back injuries frequently involve damage to the sacroiliac ligaments, and often patients are told by those proficient in manipulative medicine that their hip is "out of place." While this term is not used in conventional medicine, it is actually often correct. The weakened ligament caused by injury allows the whole ilium, or hip, to rotate around, usually making one leg longer than the other. This is fairly easy to diagnose. When these injured sacroiliac joints are treated repeatedly by manipulation but the hip won't stay in place, the ligaments have most likely been damaged. The use of prolotherapy in this instance can be exceedingly helpful.

Here is a brief description of the process of providing prolotherapy: While a variety of injection materials can be used, most often we employ a dextrose (sugar) solution of 12.5 percent or more, often coupled with a weak solution of phenol, and perhaps sodium morrhuate (a fish oil) in sterile form. These materials act as irritants to the ligaments and cause the body to start producing fibroblasts. Some of you might be surprised that dextrose can irritate the body, as it is a natural material. It is true that diluted doses of dextrose don't have an inflammatory or stimulatory effect, but once the concentration gets to 12.5 percent or more, it can take on a new role and be effective in this capacity.

We inject this solution into the ligaments we wish to stimulate, a procedure that will obviously be different for each joint of the body. The number of treatments, which can be given every two to four weeks, differs depending on the size and area of the ligaments or tendon areas that need to be stimulated. For example, an elbow problem, which most often would reflect what is commonly called *tennis elbow*, might respond to just two or three treatments. A shoulder or ankle problem usually responds to three treatments. Lower back and knee areas, which have a much larger ligamentous component, usually require six treatments or more to provide healing.

Once the materials have been injected, I urge my patients not to use any anti-inflammatory medications including aspirin, Aleve, ibuprofen in its many forms (including Advil and Motrin), or Celebrex, for the entire duration of the treatment program. If pain medication is needed, Tylenol or specific stronger pain medication can be prescribed. We recommend that patients avoid ice or heat for the first few days after injections are provided, as ice may diminish the inflammatory process we are trying to create, and heat may exacerbate it to the point that the patient may suffer needlessly.

It is very important that the physician providing these injections is also trained in manipulative medicine. It is vital that when these tissues tighten up, they tighten up correctly, anatomically. We encourage patients to use the area that we have injected as much as possible after the injections, as that helps the tissues to heal in the position of function.

Kristina's Story

Kristina was a nineteen-year-old woman referred to me by a local physiatrist who had tried for several years to get her hip to stay in place using manual medicine. He could get her hip into place, but no matter how hard he tried, it just wouldn't stay there. This physiatrist was familiar with the potential benefits of prolotherapy, and he recommended her to me for treatment. After explaining the process to Kristina and her family, I proceeded with the injections. After four treatments, each involving multiple injections of the ligaments covering the sacroiliac joints, her back held in place nicely. After years of persistent, debilitating low back pain, she became pain free for about a year.

It would be wonderful if this was the conclusion of the story in the form of a happy ending (there is one, hold on), but after a year Kristina developed severe migraine headaches, which seemed to have been set off by orthodontic procedures including the use of braces and spacers. Her orthodontist told her that her migraine headaches could not possibly have been caused by tightening her braces. Unfortunately, in my experience, this can indeed happen, and all too frequently. He referred Kristina to a neurologist who provided a variety of medications for the headaches. None of these medications worked very well and actually caused some severely limiting side effects including mental fogginess, fatigue, and even more headaches, all of which interfered with Kristina's ability to cope with schoolwork.

Eventually I put this all together and sent her to another dentist who specialized in using bracing techniques that incorporated knowledge of craniosacral mechanics (see the previous chapter). With this dentist's help, Kristina's migraines improved dramatically. However, during this time, her hips began to go out again and would not stay in place, even though we'd gotten them to do so for the whole year previous. I found that if I could get her jaw back into alignment, my hip adjustments, along with a single additional prolotherapy treatment, now held. It truly is fascinating, the ways in which certain areas of the body relate to other areas in completely unsuspected patterns. Kristina has essentially been well now for several years, without the need for additional osteopathic manipulation or prolotherapy.

Here we have a case in which the combination of prolotherapy and creative manipulative medicine has resulted in the healing that the patient has longed for.

I believe that we're going to see a lot more prolotherapy usage in the future. In the past several years, new research has revealed that much of what we used to call tendonitis is actually *tendonosis*. These words may seem similar, but they call forth a very different understanding of the mechanical causes for pain. *Tendonitis* refers to an inflammatory condition of the tendon. For many years we have treated all inflamed and tender tendons with anti-inflammatory medication and steroid injections with the presumed diagnosis of tendonitis. We have known for quite some time that repeated steroid injections may actually weaken the tendons even further, and while these treatments help some patients, they don't help a significant number of afflicted patients. New research shows that these tendons are really not inflamed, but damaged. Thus, it is reflected by the diagnostic term *tendonosis*, which means that some of the fibers of the tendons are actually weakened and torn as they insert into the bone.

This new understanding of diagnosis provides us with an innovative rationale for treatment and explains why our old treatment didn't always work very well. To heal damaged, torn tendon-insertions, prolotherapy is a much more logical approach. In fact, it is much more useful than steroid injections and works far better over the long haul. By injecting these damaged fibers and using prolotherapy to stimulate the body to lay down new fibroblasts, we create a thicker, stronger tendon. This enables us not only to heal these tissues, but to create a stronger tissue, one that would have been rendered weak by steroid injections.

My Story

Six or seven years ago, while playing basketball with my son, I jumped up with my right arm fully extended in an attempt to block his shot and experienced a pain so intense that it literally dropped me to my knees. On reflection, I recalled that I'd had some twinges of pain in that shoulder for several years, but nothing prepared me for that moment. After that initial commanding shoulder pain, things eased up a bit but then slowly and insidiously became chronic and worse. I was still able to work with that shoulder, experiencing moderate but tolerable amounts of pain, but I couldn't lift up my arm completely.

Over the next six months, I saw several of the finest osteopathic physicians I knew, and each graciously treated me. But it made no difference. I could no longer sleep on my right side, but the most frustrating part was that I couldn't put my arm around my wife as we sat on the couch to watch television or read. That is what really motivated me to get treatment.

I eventually ran into an old friend, a wonderful osteopathic physician and practitioner of prolotherapy in Columbia, Missouri, named Larry Bader. When I visited Larry, I finally received an explanation for my pain that made sense to me. He described my injury as a "weakening of the shoulder capsule," a diagnosis with which I was not familiar. Larry smiled, noting that he hadn't been either until he'd experienced the same symptoms several years before. Essentially, the weakened ligaments of my shoulder capsule had allowed the joint structures to collapse upon themselves, permitting the supraspinatus tendon to rub against the acromion, a nubbin of bone projecting downward from the scapula (shoulder blade). This is what was causing my shoulder symptoms. I have learned, subsequently, that this is actually quite a common condition, one often missed by specialists.

So I drove the three hours to Columbia, Missouri, for my three prolotherapy treatments, spaced about a month apart. While moderately painful, the injections were certainly tolerable, and I was sore for only a few days afterwards. Treatment did not interfere with my ability to work. After the third treatment, it was clear that my pain was gone, and I could sleep on my shoulder again. But I still had a somewhat frozen shoulder, and I still could not lift my arm past shoulder level toward my head. I then received several treatments by a skilled physical therapist, which freed up my shoulder, and by working and exercising that shoulder I was able to achieve complete range of motion. I have not had a lick of pain or difficulty with my shoulder in the ensuing five or six years since I received my prolotherapy injections. Had I not done prolotherapy, I am fairly certain that this condition would eventually have deteriorated into a rotator cuff problem, which would have required surgery.

Here is one more story to illustrate the potential benefits of prolotherapy. It's about yet another patient who was told that joint replacement was the only possible treatment for her symptoms.

Betty's Story

I first saw Betty in 2000, when she was sixty-one. She was concerned about a wide variety of medical problems including generalized joint pains, chronic fatigue, dizziness, hypoglycemia, psoriasis, and a recurring rectal fissure. In short, she presented to us with the typical kinds of problems that I see in my office on a daily basis. Using the Big Six/Little Six approach outlined in this book, I uncovered thyroid problems, adrenal deficiencies, bowel dysbiosis, and allergy troubles that soon led to a marked improvement in her health. She was quite happy with the excellent improvement in her health.

By late 2001, however, the deterioration of Betty's right knee joint became her central problem. Her orthopedic surgeon had recently performed arthroscopy for that knee, but she described the results of that procedure as disappointing. She was now informed by her surgeon that her right knee joint was bone-on-bone, meaning that there was no cartilage left in the knee to protect the joint. He told her in no uncertain terms that the only hope left for her would be to undergo total knee replacement.

As she was still a relatively young woman of sixty-three, she began to read up on prolotherapy and became intrigued with the possibility of this treatment for her knee. When she discovered that I could provide that service, we began treatments in early 2002. Since her knee damage was more extensive than most of my patients, it took ten prolotherapy injection sessions to produce the desired results. Betty was delighted that her pain was virtually gone; she could now walk up and down stairs without difficulty and resume the game of golf, which she had been unable to play for several years.

Seven years later, Betty has required no additional prolotherapy treatments, and she continues to do well. She is thrilled to have avoided knee replacement surgery for so many years, and although we cannot be certain that this surgery will never be necessary, there is no sign currently that she is anywhere near that possibility.

Like Betty, I have often found that many patients who have been told, "There's nothing more we can do for you," have responded beautifully to prolotherapy and had much or all of their pain relieved. Please keep in mind that this is not a panacea for the treatment of all pain. It is specifically designed to treat pain that is caused by weakened or damaged ligaments and tendons. As you can see, when used properly, it can be of enormous healing benefit.

Further Reading

Cyriax, J H., and P J. Cyriax. *Cyriax's Illustrated Manual of Orthopaedic Medicine*. 2nd ed. Oxford: Butterworth/Heinemann, 1993.

Dorman, Thomas A., and Thomas H. Ravin. *Diagnosis and Injection Techniques in Orthopedic Medicine*. Baltimore: Williams & Wilkins, 1991.

Hackett, George S. *Ligament and Tendon Relaxation Treated By Prolotherapy*. 3rd ed. Springfield, IL: C. C. Thomas, 1991.

Other Concepts and Treatments

*C*ongratulations! You have just made it through advanced biochemistry. With the completion of the "Big Six" and "Little Six" areas of investigation, we have a wonderful beginning for our understanding of the causes of most chronic illness, which simultaneously provides us with a clear treatment approach.

This book was always intended to be one of hope, a place where patients can come to search for their next helpful step. Out of the many, many alternative treatments and concepts available to us, I am selecting just a few subjects for additional discussion. These subjects are chosen for their importance to many patients.

Countless individuals are afflicted with atherosclerosis and the subsequent blockages of vital arteries, including the coronary arteries that supply the heart with blood, the carotid arteries that supply the brain with blood, and the peripheral arteries that supply the extremities with blood. Statistically, this is the most common cause of death in America. For those patients who have not benefited sufficiently from conventional approaches, the use of chelation therapy may be just what the doctor ordered. Chapter 19 provides a preliminary discussion of this underused treatment.

Cancer is the second most common cause of death in our society, and, when advanced, can be a serious source of suffering for patients and their families. Alternative concepts and approaches for the treatment of cancer are presented in Chapter 21, along with a similar discussion on the treatment options for the related issues of autoimmune disease.

The newly identified epidemic of autism is a frightening subject for all new parents, and I wanted to bring to your attention the exciting and effective approaches to understanding and treating autism, which are offered in Chapter 22.

Chapter 19

Chelation

The Bind That Ties

Much is written about chelation, and as with any controversial therapy, much of this information is prone to misunderstanding and strong opinion. Since the primary use of chelation is for treating arterial blockage from atherosclerosis, most of the objections to its use come from cardiologists. They have come to believe that there is inadequate scientific evidence to confirm its value, while ignoring the existence of medical books entirely devoted to providing this evidence. As this conflicting information brings us to a bit of an impasse, let us explore this subject in more detail.

The word *chelation* simply means "to bind," coming from the root word, *chela,* which is Greek for "claw." In general, the materials being bound are minerals, especially toxic heavy metals such as mercury, lead, aluminum, cadmium, tin, and arsenic, among others. Usually, when patients talk about chelation, they are referring to the use of *ethylene diamine tetra-acetic acid* (EDTA) chelation. This is by far the commonest form of chelation currently in use, and it utilizes this chemical to bind to heavy metals, especially lead, to pull them out of the body. The chelating agent, in this case EDTA, binds tighter to the metal than body tissues do. The body then eliminates the EDTA with the heavy metal attached, moving it through the kidneys and out of the body through the urine. This has long been recognized by conventional medicine as the treatment of choice for lead toxicity.

EDTA chelation first became available during World War II, when it was used to detoxify workers who had excessive exposure to lead-based paints, most commonly from their work in the shipyards, where large quantities of these paints would be sprayed without adequate ventilation. It was discovered, however, that several workers with coronary heart obstruction (angina), had significant relief of their heart symptoms when their lead toxicity was treated with EDTA, intravenously. Astute physicians who observed this wondered if EDTA might successfully treat other patients with coronary arterial blockages, and, to their surprise, it did. This launched the concept of "chelation" treatments in the management of arterial blockage from cholesterol plaques.

An EDTA treatment is fairly simple. We mix up a sterile intravenous bag that contains an exact amount of EDTA, one that is calculated by precise measurement of the patient's kidney function. Added to the EDTA are magnesium and usually additional materials that may include small amounts of heparin, potassium, sodium bicarbonate, procaine, vitamin C, and B vitamins. The main limiting factor as to how much EDTA can be given is how well the kidneys work. Before we start the chelation process, we obtain a twenty-four-hour urine collection coupled with a blood test that measures the creatinine clearance, considered the most accurate way to define how well the kidneys are filtering. A normal creatinine clearance is 80 to 120 cc/min. Anything lower than this range indicates that the dosage of EDTA must be decreased so as not to overload the kidneys.

With the correct amount of materials, the patient receives a series of twenty or more intravenous sessions, initially given once or twice per week. Each of these sessions lasts an average of three hours. Depending on clinical response, these treatments can continue until maximum improvement has occurred. What I typically see is that patients report fewer episodes of angina, less shortness of breath, improved energy, an overall improvement in their sense of well being, lower blood pressure, and a decreased need for their cardiac medications.

At this point, we continue these intravenous treatments once every four to six weeks as maintenance therapy indefinitely. We have discovered that if the patient goes more than six months without receiving treatments, some of the benefits may disappear. From the relief of carotid arterial blockages, I have personally seen fairly dramatic improvements in cardiac function, improved blood flow to the feet and legs from the relief of peripheral artery disease, and improved blood flow to the brain. These treatments are *safe*. In twenty-five years of providing thousands of these treatments, I've only observed a few minor side effects and nothing negative of any significance. That's not a bad track record, especially when we compare it to the conventional medical alternative of surgery. There are well known, life-threatening complications of that surgery, and the benefits may be short-lived. Balloon angioplasties often do not last for long, and stints often become blocked. While I don't believe that chelation is for everyone, it is certainly an option for many. Let's put it this way: if I were personally diagnosed for any coronary blockage, I would get chelated before I would undergo cardiac catheterization or surgery.

As previously noted, chelation has been accompanied by intense controversy over the years. Most conventional physicians believe that this treatment has no validity whatsoever and should never be attempted. Other physicians who have observed the effects of these treatments are convinced that this is a safe and effective process. As I write these words, several large ongoing clinical trials are in place, attempting to clarify the answer to these important questions. Some observers of this controversy boil it down to economics: when you can charge $40,000 for a highly technical cardiac procedure, why would you consider an approach that only nets you $2,000? Many patients who have benefited greatly from this procedure have been quick to point out this discrepancy.

Duncan's Story

Duncan first came to me when he was fifty-nine, in February 1997. He expressed his concern very succinctly at our first visit: "I've got plugged up arteries." Duncan related a long history of coronary artery disease that began in 1980, when he underwent a six-vessel bypass procedure. Then, in 1992, he had a second four-vessel procedure performed. He had become concerned with increasing symptoms of shortness of breath and chest tightness, with an angiogram performed in December 1996 showing 100 percent occlusion of his right coronary artery grafts and 75 to 90 percent occlusion of a second graft area. His cardiologist did not feel that he could reach that area of occlusion with a balloon or stint, and medications were not effective in improving his condition.

I began treating Duncan with EDTA chelation therapy, which involved twenty initial treatments and one treatment monthly thereafter. Duncan did extremely well with his program, noting marked improvement clinically, which was confirmed a year later on follow-up angiogram. By the time he had completed the first ten treatments, he was no longer short of breath, no longer had chest pain, and was able to go to work all day with increased stamina and energy. His cardiologist was amazed by his improvement, but as is usually the case, was loath to attribute this improvement to Duncan's chelational efforts.

Duncan did very well on this program, and he was able to continue full-time work for many years until his expected retirement at age sixty-five. He continued his treatments but did have a minor setback in 2007, when he needed the placement of two stints by his cardiologist. Two years later, continuing his chelation treatments, Duncan continues to be active and healthy and is convinced that he would not be alive today had he not undergone this form of treatment. I suspect that is true. Although his cardiologist still doubts the benefit of his chelation treatments, he has often commented to Duncan that his impressive improvement is baffling and admits that it cannot be explained by conventional medical concepts. But Duncan just smiles and shakes his head; he has no intention of stopping this treatment that has proven so effective.

Again, I often hear from conventional cardiologists that there is no evidence of chelation's efficacy, but there is actually quite a bit of it. It depends, really, on what you read. If you don't read any alternative medical literature, it's not surprising that you're not aware of this evidence and information. Much of this book discusses what I would consider cutting edge medical concepts, so my own opinions are based more on what I have observed and seen with my own eyes rather than on the opinions of others. But please don't misunderstand, for I highly value the opinions of my colleagues and will take the time to listen closely to what they have to say. However, often those opinions are based on a theoretical understanding of an idea, rather than direct hands-on experience with a particular treatment, and it is the latter that I especially value.

There is a clear distinction between theory and practice—while theories are nice, how real, live patients respond to treatments is what I really care about. That's the front line of medical practice: helping patients. If you spend any time around a group of patients that have had chelation treatments, it is difficult to walk away from that experience without being impressed. It is commonplace for patients to receive these three-hour infusions in small groups in my office, and listening to them recount their experiences to each other makes it difficult to discard these consistently reported benefits. After twenty-five years of administering these treatments, I am convinced that they have great value, and I would estimate that 80 percent of the patients who have participated would agree.

Melvin's Story

Sixty-two-year-old Melvin first came to my office in 2003. He had undergone a five-vessel bypass procedure fifteen years previously and originally came to me for persistent left-side numbness and tingling over his entire left rib cage, radiating up into his left neck area. He had been extensively evaluated in several medical centers, with no explanation for his symptoms. I eventually treated him with osteopathic manipulation, which over the course of many months, resulted in virtually complete resolution of his symptoms.

But in January 2005, Melvin had a mild heart attack and had several stints placed by his cardiologist. He was placed on the medication Plavix, which is standard procedure following the placements of stints. The side effects of the Plavix were almost worse than the cardiac symptoms: severe, sudden episodes of esophageal spasm that kept putting Melvin in the hospital for evaluation. And the stints just kept on coming. Over the next year, Melvin had ten procedures with the placement of a total of fifteen stints, performed on an almost monthly basis!

Despite the fact that he lived a considerable distance from our office, I encouraged Melvin to begin chelation to avert the continuation of this process. He agreed, although the procedure was difficult for him, as he experienced the very unusual side effect of shaking for several hours after each infusion. But as long as he continued his chelation, he was able to do well and did not require additional stinting. After approximately eight months of treatments, he elected to stop them, and within a few months he was back requiring stinting procedures at an alarming frequency. The benefits of chelation therapy in this case seemed very clear to me, and they did to Melvin, as well.

The second most common form of chelation is the one we use for mercury toxicity (See Chapter 10). It is only recently that we learned how to accurately measure chronic mercury exposure, and as most physicians and dentists don't seem to realize that this is much of a problem, they do not address it. I can understand why dentists would rather not accept this information, as they have been placing mercury amalgam fillings in our mouths for over sixty years. It would be difficult for any health practitioner to believe that what she has been doing could be harmful, but as our knowledge grows, for many patients this seems to be the case.

We consider that there are three major sources of mercury exposure: fish ingestion, the emissions from coal-burning plants, and leakage from our dental amalgam fillings. Of those, most experts working in this field believe that the amalgams represent our greatest exposure. This does not mean that you have to run out and get your fillings removed today. Just because you have them doesn't mean they've leaked mercury into your body. Removing fillings is expensive and painful, and it should be done in a very specific manner by specially trained dentists so that additional toxicity does not occur. If you have reasons to suspect mercury toxicity (see the list of symptoms in Chapter 10), get your mercury levels checked using the DMPS challenge test, described later in this chapter.

Natalie's Story

Natalie, at sixty years of age, presented to my office three years ago. She was concerned about her hormonal balance, having been on Prempro and other synthetic hormones previously. However, those materials did not agree with her, and since she was hearing a great deal about the potential toxicities of synthetic hormones, she was fearful of taking them. Natalie was especially worried about her memory, focus, and concentration, and had particular concerns about her ability to work with numbers. This was of great importance in her job as a bank supervisor. For many years, she had prided herself on her ability to keep track of multiple columns of numbers at will, and now she could barely keep it straight. Natalie also reported a significant drop in energy, as well as hair loss and emotional instability. She could now cry at the drop of a hat and felt at times like she could "tear someone's head off."

Upon examination, I found that Natalie had a low DHEA level, so I started her on 25 mg DHEA each morning. We discovered, as well, that she had low levels of estrogen and progesterone, so we provided a small dose of those bioidentical hormones. Both low estrogen and low DHEA levels are often associated with decreased cognitive function, but even after using those supplements for several months, Natalie was only slightly better from a cognitive standpoint. While her energy was quite a bit better and her mood much improved, her biggest concern was still that she couldn't think clearly, especially in working with numbers. When I performed the DMPS challenge test, however, I found her to have a significant elevation in her mercury levels. We then began a monthly series of DMPS intravenous treatments, providing a total of eight. This was followed by the use of oral DMSA for the next year, and also followed by the removal of her mercury amalgam fillings by a knowledgeable biological dentist. Slowly and steadily, within that year, the vast majority of her cognitive facilities returned, and she was now functioning much better at work and at home, and very pleased with her improvement. Natalie feels that she is back to her old self, and that improvement has held steady over the ensuing years.

Mercury tends to accumulate in our tissues, especially in the brain, and once there, it binds so strongly to those tissues that it is hard to remove it. Time alone does very little. We have learned that simply measuring mercury levels in the blood, urine, hair, or stool will not reveal its presence, as it is tightly bound to body tissues. In order to diagnose it, therefore, we have to use a chelating agent (in this case DMPS is considered the best by most authorities on the subject). The chelator (DMPS) binds tighter to the mercury than it does to body tissues and, again, pulls it out through the kidneys. By providing an infusion of intravenous DMPS over fifteen minutes, and then collecting the patient's urine for twenty-four hours and sending it out to our reference laboratory for analysis, we can get an accurate estimate of the mercury content of the tissues. This is an elegant and accurate test. This, too, is cutting-edge medicine, and experts are not in complete agreement about the best way to measure and treat mercury toxicity. What I have discussed represents a consensus of our current thinking, but some physicians prefer an oral chelator called DMSA, and others use the medication penicillamine. The point of this discussion is not to provide the definitive answer as to how to measure and treat mercury toxicity but rather to suggest that this is an often missed diagnosis and should be considered as a possible contributing factor for anyone who is ill and for whom no clear answers to cause of their illness have been uncovered.

We have discovered several hundred patients with mercury toxicity, and most of them would tell you that removing the mercury has been of great benefit in their recovery. Newer forms of administration of chelating materials have been recently proposed, including oral, rectal, and transdermal administration. Unfortunately, there is very little evidence to suggest that these routes of administration work anywhere near as well as the intravenous materials. Patients are thrilled to hear that they might not need to take the expensive and time-consuming IVs, but at this time I cannot recommend the oral or other newer forms as an acceptable alternative.

Further Reading

Cranton, Elmer M. *Bypassing Bypass Surgery: Chelation Therapy: A Non-surgical Treatment for Reversing Arteriosclerosis, Improving Blocked Circulation, and Slowing the Aging Process.* Charlottesville, VA: Hampton Roads, 2001.

McDonagh, E.W. and C.J. Rudolph. *A Collection of Published Papers Showing the Efficacy of EDTA Chelation Therapy.* Gladstone, MD: McDonagh Medical Center, 1991.

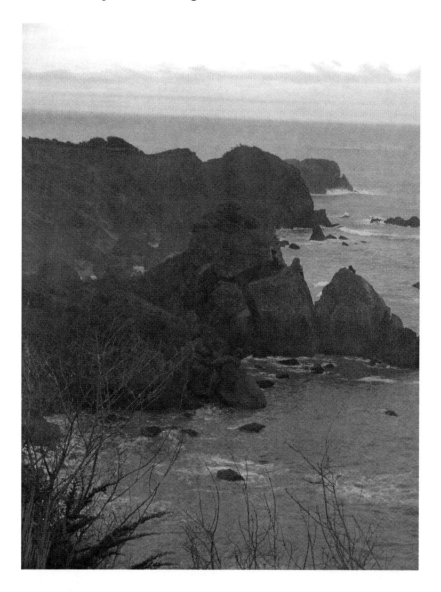

Chapter 20

Breech Version

One Good Turn Deserves Another

When I was younger, I was led to believe that the Great Gods of Science and Medicine were demanding but fair. If you conducted meticulous research and followed the prescribed statistical methods to analyze the data, and if you could then prove that you had uncovered some new aspect of the Truth, then those gods would smile upon you and reward your sacrifices of time and energy and hard work by embracing this new information, and everyone would live happily ever after. Boy, was I naïve. What I had not understood was that the Great Gods of Science and Medicine were in fact human beings. And human beings, flawed as they are, are not prone to embrace change. We say we do, but when push comes to shove, most of us really like things as they are, and we resist change intensely. It is our resistance to change that is the Truth; planting the seeds of new information into hostile soil requires many years of persistence before that soil begins to allow those seeds to evolve. Alas, sometimes those seeds never even germinate.

Please understand that what I'm talking about here is the emergence of new ideas or concepts, not about new drugs or technologies. Yes, we embrace new drugs and technologies immediately, sometimes too readily. Often the public confuses this industry-driven innovation with the way in which ideas are integrated into the body of information we call *medicine*.

Let me make clear that what the public assumes, incorrectly, is that all physicians are trained in and believe in a uniform body of information called Medicine, which is taught at all medical schools. No such entity exists. Each medical school is strongly under the influence of several of its more renowned senior members, experts who insert their personal views into the curriculum of their particular school. Thus, each institution has its own body of information, which is somewhat similar to, yet significantly different from, the material that is taught in other schools. That is why those of you who have been to several different physicians are surprised to discover that these doctors don't agree with each other about many aspects of your diagnosis and treatment. And why should they? Each of them most likely trained under different experts in different medical schools.

When I practiced in Minnesota, the two major medical schools in the area were the Mayo Clinic, in Rochester, and the University of Minnesota, in the Twin Cities of Minneapolis and St. Paul. As I practiced in Duluth, I found that many conversations with physicians, the majority of whom had trained in one of those two excellent institutions, often boiled down to them saying, "We always do it this way at Mayo" or "this is the way it was done at The U." There was little ground for cross discussion between them.

In this chapter, I would like to share my personal journey down the path of research. It thankfully occurred relatively early in my career and helped me to understand how information is either integrated into or rejected by conventional medicine. It was a real eye-opener. Although some of this research may seem a bit detailed and of a different ilk than what I have presented in the rest of this book, what I am trying to convey is a story about the bigger picture. If you can understand the larger ramifications of how new information is processed by conventional medicine (and usually rejected or shelved for indeterminate periods of time), then much of the rest of this book will make a great deal more sense.

This particular research story is about babies that are lying in their mother's uterus with their bottoms pointed down into the pelvis, which we call the *breech position*.

The vast majority of babies lie in the uterus with their heads down, toward the pelvis. We call this the *vertex position* because in medicine the vertex is our name for the crown or top of the head. Sometimes, for reasons still not entirely clear, the baby finds itself in the breech position, a variation from the normal vertex. This is not uncommon in the early stages of pregnancy, but as gestation proceeds, the babies tend to turn spontaneously into the far more common vertex position. However, research shows that after thirty-six weeks of pregnancy (keeping in mind that forty weeks are what we consider to be a normal term pregnancy), only 5 percent will turn by themselves, a process which we call *breech version*. The word *version* simply means "turn." The reason this is important is that breech babies are at higher risks for complications of labor and delivery, and because of that, many more Caesarian sections are done to make their delivery safer. If it were possible to *turn* those babies physically so they were head-down, or in the vertex position, it would be much safer for both mother and child and would decrease the known complications of breech delivery or Caesarian section. Physically turning a breech baby has been tried in the past with some success, usually by administering medications to relax the uterus and using some degree of force to move the baby about. Unfortunately, that approach was found to be associated with significant risks of damage to both mother and baby, and those risks were regarded as unacceptable.

In 1976, while practicing in Mendocino, California, I was doing a fair amount of obstetrics as part of my practice. A young, pregnant mother came into the office one day, and she was visibly quite distraught. She had felt her baby in the breech position and knew what that meant: a possible Caesarian section. She had gotten so anxious about that possibility that she could hardly function. I really had no idea what to do for her, but she was so worried that I had her lie down on my examination table, and I placed her in a particular position of relaxation that I'd learned in my study of Reichian therapy (emotional release work). While lying on her back, with her knees bent and slightly apart, I asked her to take deep breaths. She did this for ten or fifteen minutes, during which time her legs shook intensely, and the shaking spread to other parts of her body. I encouraged that she allow herself to do this, to not resist the trembling process, which is what most people naturally tend to do if they don't understand what is happening. This patient needed to utilize the immense value of shaking in assisting her body to release its accumulated tensions. She shook rather intensely during this process, and when she got up off the table, she was quite excited and gave me a big hug. I was a little taken aback by this, as it didn't seem that we'd done all that much. Yes, she was more relaxed, but certainly not deserving of this amount of elation.

Seeing my reaction, she asked, "Didn't you see the baby turn?" Since I wasn't looking for it, I hadn't. I had examined the baby's position before we started, and it was indeed breech. When I rechecked her, the baby was back in the preferred vertex position. Wow! She delivered her baby uneventfully several weeks later. However, what happened on that exam table intrigued me. Was this process something we could use for other women with breech presentations? Or was it just a coincidence? It seemed easy enough to find out.

I asked my colleagues who were doing obstetrics to refer to me their breech presentations that had reached thirty-six weeks' gestation. My plan was to repeat this process of shaking-induced relaxation with just a few patients in order to see if I could rule out coincidence. As this was a small-town practice, I saw only a total of eight patients over the next few years, but six of them turned from the breech into the vertex position. As I began to research the probability of this happening, it was clear that this was unlikely to be mere chance. I was also aware that for my profession to take these observations seriously, I would need to attempt this on a lot more patients so that the statistics would be meaningful. I was under the impression at that time that a properly done research project with well-done statistics was sufficient to change the way my colleagues thought.

So several years later, I moved to Duluth, Minnesota, where I became the assistant director of a Family Practice Residency Program and had access to many more patients. Although it took quite a bit of convincing, I eventually got my colleagues to refer their breech presentations to me, and I worked my way up to fifty-five consecutive patients. By this point, the simple technique had proven to be very safe, with no observed negative consequences, which were carefully sought. Forty percent of these babies turned spontaneously. Left alone, without treatment, only 5 percent of these babies would have turned on their own. In the world of statistics, this had a p value of $<.001$, which is considered by experts to mean that the odds of this happening by chance are about one in a thousand. This technique, by rigorous scientific standards, was proven to be valid and useful. We had circumvented the need for a Caesarian section and all that entails in an additional 35 percent of our patients.

I was quite excited by this and was invited to present my research findings formally by the American Academy of Family Practice and later at a regional meeting of the American College of Gynecology and Obstetrics. At both conferences, my work was well received, but to my surprise, what I repeatedly heard from attendees of the meetings was, "I see the data but I don't believe it." One of my colleagues even took the time to learn the method, and he tried it on a dozen patients with identical results, publishing his findings in a small medical journal. My osteopathic mentor, Dr. James Jealous, later showed that specific osteopathic manipulation techniques for the cervix and uterus, performed very gently, accomplished the same results. This leads me to believe that the breech position often represents the manifestation of an excessive amount of tension in the pelvis, so much so that the baby finds itself without enough *room* to turn on its own. From the results of my research, it seems logical to assert that if we can alter this pelvic tension by getting the tissues to relax, the baby would now have sufficient room to turn itself into the head down position. I suspect that a combination of this relaxation technique with osteopathic manipulation might prove to have even better results, and that is for future researchers to explore.

Most fascinating to me at that time was the reception of this research by my profession, which really took me aback. I had spent years doing this work and generating research data that was quite impressive, only to find a cold response. I had labored under the delusion that "if you prove it, they will believe," only to find that this was not true. The truth, which took me quite a lot of time to accept, was that changing belief takes a lot more than one well-done study. As I have suggested, doctors are just people, and people find it very hard to change what they believe no matter how carefully you present that information. This was a real eye-opener for me, and although disappointing, it helped me wake up to the realization that not everything we believe is true, and that I might have to do some digging on my own to figure things out. So I did.

I hope you have noticed by now that this book is about all the valuable, practical ideas and treatments that have enabled thousands of my patients to heal and to improve their health. Many of these ideas have not yet been embraced by conventional medicine, but I am not alone. There is a growing body of physicians who agree with these concepts and have also applied them to their own clinical practice with similar results.

Under the sometimes false guise of science, currently utilizing the name of *evidence-based medicine,* we are in danger of distancing ourselves from a whole body of useful information generated by many talented and perceptive physicians who have gone back to the time-honored process of learning about their patients and simply making observations about what works. Treating those patients that conventional medicine has essentially given up on, using our best intentions coupled with new medical information and new diagnostic tools, we do our best to alleviate suffering and pain. And mostly we succeed.

We have tried to come to an understanding with this new medical god, Evidence-Based Medicine, and to realize its limitations. Since conventional medicine has not obtained much "evidence" about these newer ideas, either pro or con, it chooses to ignore this new body of information entirely. It may take many years until it can formulate its own opinion. And at the rate we're going, a lot of patients may remain undiagnosed and untreated for a really long time. Right now, we have millions of struggling patients with nowhere to turn for help. How can we ignore their needs and hide behind the weak excuse that these ideas have not been proven to everyone's satisfaction? By now you will understand that the long-standing differences of medical opinion which have always existed are not so easily resolved and are rarely resolved to any physician's personal satisfaction.

The most common questions about this material from my patients are, "Why don't my other doctors know about this?" and "Why don't my other doctors think this information is of value?" I cannot, of course, speak to the question of why an individual physician has a certain belief. I have attempted, throughout this book, to explain how this happens, since I believe it is very important that we understand these philosophical differences. These differences translate into profoundly different paths of diagnosis and treatment.

Chapter 21

Alternative Approaches to Cancer and Autoimmune Diseases

Dr. Livingston, I Presume?

*D*espite billions of research dollars and the efforts of countless dedicated scientists, we have made only a small amount of progress in the treatment of cancer. In fact, even with newer and more sophisticated diagnostic equipment, the incidence of many cancers continues to increase at an alarming rate. How can this occur? The answer, I suspect, is that our understanding of how the body develops cancer is inadequate. Thus, we must return to a recurring mantra of this book: without a clear grasp of the cause(s), how can we possibly refine the treatments?

Conventional Treatments of Cancer

The current conventional treatment of cancer involves three major considerations: surgery, chemotherapy, and radiation. In fact, in certain states, there are actually laws that limit all treatments to those options alone. These treatments certainly have their place, and many forms of cancer are eradicated by their proper use. But first, we must try to understand the causes.

We do know something about the factors that allow a body to develop cancer. One of these factors is our genetic structure: we carry certain genes that, if activated, interfere with the proper workings of our immune system. Let me emphasize the phrase, "if activated." This means that even if you have inherited genes that may contribute to the creation of cancer, they may never come into play. There is credible evidence that proper diet and lifestyle can prevent this activation from happening.

The healthy functionality of our immune system is the key to preventing and treating cancer. We have an elaborate surveillance system in which special cells within our body are constantly looking for anything foreign, anything that is "not us." If these special cells find abnormal cells that do not perfectly resemble the cell lines with which they are familiar, they either destroy them on the spot, or call for reinforcements to do the job. Sometimes they mistakenly identify our normal cells as being something foreign, to be attacked, and when that happens we are attacking ourselves, which we call *autoimmunity*. We will discuss this in more detail later in this chapter.

It is generally believed that we constantly generate abnormal, cancerous cells within our bodies, and that our immune system is rapidly identifying and destroying those cells. When that process breaks down or gets compromised, cancer develops. By definition, a growing cancer means that our immune system has not been able to deal with these abnormal cells properly.

At this point, in conventional medicine, we treat the growing cancer first by surgically excising it, if that is technically possible. Depending on the exact nature of the tumor, we may decide that surgery alone is sufficient treatment, or that additional treatment in the form of chemotherapy or radiation is necessary to eradicate the tumor. Keep in mind that there are many types of cancer, which are usually named after the cell-line and organ from which it grows, and each type is biologically different from the next.

But here's where it can get a little dicey. Both chemotherapy and radiation are destructive treatments that are capable of both destroying the cancer and damaging the immune system. I view them as double-edged swords—while they may be life-saving, they may also interfere with the functions of the immune system that ultimately are necessary for healing. Making the decision to accept chemotherapy or radiation can, therefore, be quite difficult, and it requires an intimate knowledge about not only the biology of the specific cancer in question, but also the strength of the individual patient's immune system at that moment in time.

Basically, treating cancer is in some ways similar to treating an infection. While most people believe that infections are cured by the antibiotics they take, this is not really true. The antibiotic, if properly prescribed (keeping in mind that we don't have treatment available for most viral infections), will indeed kill off a large number of microorganisms, but not all of them. It is our immune system that must come into play to finish the job. The same is true for treating cancer: if we can lower the number of abnormal cells in our body using surgery, radiation, or chemotherapy, then we can increase the likelihood that our immune system will be able to get on top of the situation and finish the job of killing these abnormal cells. But if in the process of treatment we have damaged the key system needed for healing, how are we to heal? That is the tricky part, and you should begin to see how difficult it can be for physicians and patients to make these decisions.

Having said all this, please do not lose sight of the fact that this discussion has not begun to include the concept of the cause(s) of cancer, without which more specific treatment cannot be delivered. I believe that this is the major weakness in our approach to cancer today. We spend billions of dollars to refine our surgical procedures and to develop more effective radiation approaches and new chemotherapy drugs. This is well and good, but it doesn't move us any closer to getting to cause, and without that information, I suspect, we cannot make the kind of progress necessary to really make significant inroads to the cure of this disease.

Worse, the industry that cancer treatment has become actually resists the influx of new ideas by invoking the time-honored tradition of claiming they are "unproven" and hence potentially dangerous to patients. While I am not advocating the indiscriminate use of unorthodox treatments, the history of cancer treatment is filled with exciting possibilities that are never given even a hint of a true test by the established medical authorities, and this is to the great detriment of the public.

As entire books have been devoted to this subject, I do not intend to bring all of these treatments to your attention in this one chapter. I would like, however, to discuss one specific approach with which I am quite familiar, and to outline several of the more well documented treatments. Once again, my goal here is to provide hope that even if you've been told that nothing else can be done, there may indeed be quite a lot that can still be done. I want to point you in those directions.

The Livingston Vaccines

I had the privilege to be the medical director of the Livingston Foundation Medical Center in San Diego from 1991 to 1995. It was there that I learned firsthand of the remarkable research and treatment created by Dr. Virginia Livingston. The story of my experiences at this facility will serve as an excellent example of what I am trying to convey about understanding the cause of cancer.

In 1947, Dr. Virginia Livingston (then Virginia Wuerthele Caspe) held the position of a school physician in New Jersey. While working there, she examined a nurse who had been diagnosed as having Raynaud's disease, a vascular condition in which the fingertips change color and become numb in response to cold temperatures. Livingston found ulcerations on the tips of several fingers, hypersensitivity along the nerves of the patient's arms and legs, and a perforation of the nasal septum, which surprisingly looked a lot like leprosy, a disease with which Livingston was familiar. These findings implied that this nurse actually had scleroderma, an autoimmune disease which often expresses itself as a severe form of Raynaud's syndrome, and this diagnosis was subsequently confirmed by biopsy. Intrigued by the similarities of the patient's symptoms to leprosy, Dr. Livingston made smears from the base of the woman's fingertip ulcers and nasal areas, and then stained them with an acid-fast dye commonly used to diagnose tuberculosis, a bacterium in the same family as leprosy. To Livingston's surprise, and that of her colleagues, the acid-fast stained cells were positive for this family of microorganisms. She treated the nurse with antibiotics known to kill these bacteria, and she recovered completely.

Intrigued by these unusual findings, Dr. Livingston took this one step further: she grew cultures of these bacteria and injected them into chicks and guinea pigs. Most of the animals became diseased; almost all of the chicks died, and the guinea pigs developed hard areas of their skin similar to what we would find in scleroderma. Some of these areas appeared cancerous, which was quite curious since the incidence of cancer in guinea pigs is very low (1 in 500,000 animals). This suggested to Livingston that scleroderma might actually be caused by these bacteria and might represent a type of slow-growing cancer. She began to screen her cancer patients with this same cell staining technique and found similar microorganisms in most of them.

Livingston published her initial findings in 1947, and those findings were later confirmed by several researchers at the Pasteur Institute in Brussels, and again confirmed by Alan Cantwell, M.D., a dermatologist in Los Angeles who published several papers in reputable journals showing the same results. Other researchers became excited about this work, and several prominent scientists joined Livingston in publishing a series of papers demonstrating the presence of these bacteria in cancer patients. As she and her colleagues investigated further, they realized that these bacteria had pleomorphic properties (meaning that they could change shape and appearance), and they were named *Progenitor cryptocides*, which is Greek for "the hidden killer." In 1949, Dr. Livingston was named head of the new Rutgers-Presbyterian Hospital Laboratory for the Study of Proliferative Diseases. She received grants from the American Cancer Society, *Reader's Digest*, Charles Pfizer and company, Lederle Laboratories, the Abbott Company, and other foundations. She was ready to begin her research in earnest.

At this time, and still today, it was generally believed that cancer was caused by a virus and not a bacterium. Over the next ten years, Livingston and her fellow researchers were able to demonstrate clearly and publish data showing that virtually every type of animal and human cancer contained these bacteria, which were similar in structure to tuberculosis and leprosy. The most striking characteristic of these bacteria was that of pleomorphism: the shape-changing capacities of these organisms presented as viral-like bodies in the tumors, which evolved after several months into larger mycoplasma-like L-forms (Mycoplasma organisms are infective germs between the size of viruses and bacteria), and then into bacterial rods and filaments. Other forms of the bacterium were also noted, including larger cysts and spore forms almost reminiscent in appearance to fungi. This means that a simple glance at these bacteria under the microscope might demonstrate a completely different appearance at different times and under different conditions. This makes these bacteria very difficult to categorize. Strains of these bacteria were sent to a number of laboratories for identification, but none could really classify them. They were something unknown and new.

With this exciting new concept that the cause of cancer might be this unusual bacterium, Livingston and company embarked on an attempt to prove it, using the time-honored concept called Koch's Postulates. This system has been used by medicine for decades to prove that a particular infectious agent causes a particular disease. Koch's Postulates are four:

1. The microorganism must be present in every case of the disease.
2. It must be possible to culture the microorganism outside the host (i.e. animal) in some artificial culture medium.
3. The inoculation of this culture into a susceptible animal must produce the disease in question.
4. The microorganism must then be able to be found in the inoculated animals and re-cultured.

By 1950, Livingston's team was able to demonstrate that the *Progenitor cryptocides* indeed fulfilled these criteria, so they published their findings in the *American Journal of the Medical Sciences*, a prominent publication, to a mixed reception. Some scientists were intrigued with this new information, but others tended to dismiss it out of hand because it was not in alignment with the viral theories that were more popular at that time.

Turning to human cancers, Dr. Livingston found that in breast cancer, positive cultures for this bacterium could be directly grown from the blood and lymph glands of cancer patients as well as from the tumors themselves. She began to feel that cancer was not simply a localized disease, confined to a single area of the patient's body, but rather a systemic, generalized disease.

As the research proceeded, Livingston became aware of a study that had preceded hers by many years. Similar work had apparently been done by George Clark, a pathologist who in 1920 reported on his successful culturing of a bacterium known as *Glover's cancer organism*. He injected this bacterium into animals, which resulted in the presence of metastasizing tumors. Livingston took this several steps further: she developed a vaccine against the *Progenitor cryptocides* bacterium and demonstrated that she could *protect* animals from getting cancer, even after they were infected by this bacterium, as long they had previously received her vaccine.

Eleanor Alexander-Jackson, a noted expert in tuberculosis and a co-investigator with Dr. Livingston in her research work, developed breast cancer in 1951. Eleanor underwent radical mastectomy surgery, but then elected to take the vaccine Livingston's team had developed from the *Progenitor cryptocides* bacterium as her follow-up treatment. The other options presented to her were more extensive surgery, cobalt radiation, or chemotherapy, all of which were urged. But Eleanor decided to go with the vaccine instead. She remained cancer-free for more than thirty years after.

However, the vaccine remained only a research tool until 1965, when a close friend of Livingston pleaded with her to help her husband. The man was diagnosed as having a large lymphoma involving the thymus gland, and he was told it was inoperable because it had already grown into the surrounding tissues. His physicians held out little hope for him. While reluctant, Dr. Livingston agreed to provide him with the vaccine. The patient responded with a complete remission of his cancer and no recurrence over twenty additional years of follow-up.

This seminal event sparked the opening of the Livingston Foundation Medical Center, founded in San Diego, California. Although Dr. Livingston died in 1990, her work continued at the clinic until several years ago, when the clinic was disbanded. However, her vaccines and other treatment materials are still available today from Dr. Edwin McClelland at the San Diego Immunotherapy Clinic, which is unfortunately the only clinic still providing this treatment.

The reason I've taken the time to relate this story is because it details the availability of solid medical research and proven therapeutic results, which are still not a part of conventional thinking or treatment. In a 1990 paper, P. B. Macomber asserts that

> Only a small number of cancer researchers today believe that bacteria play an essential role in the cancer process. Over the years, those few workers who have carried out research supporting this concept have generally been ignored or discredited. As a result, virtually no discussion of their work can be found in any modern textbook of oncology. Yet collectively, their research indicates that cell wall deficient bacteria are probably constantly associated with animal and human can-

cers, that these bacteria appear capable of inducing cancer in animals and that immunity to these bacteria sometimes protects experimental animals against certain forms of cancer.

Here's what makes this information so exciting: here we have a safe, non-toxic material, a vaccine that appears actually to address one of the causes of cancer by stimulating the immune system to improve its own ability to keep this bacterium in check. Isn't this a less drastic solution than chemotherapy or radiation?

At this point you are probably wondering whether the vaccine really worked. It did. Having worked in this clinic for more than four years with hundreds of patients with cancer and autoimmune disease, I can attest to its effectiveness. Like any treatment, it works best if used earlier in the course of disease. If we could catch patients with breast cancer or colon cancer or brain malignancies early on, we had a superb treatment response. If patients came to us when they were at death's doorstep, we didn't do very well. But even then, we were able to cure or help from 15 to 20 percent of those unfortunate individuals, all of whom had already been told by their physicians, "There's nothing more we can do for you." Once again, here was hope, slim at times, but still hope that healing or recovery was still possible.

You don't need to take my word for the effectiveness of this treatment. In 1992, The *New England Journal of Medicine* published a study in which Dr. Barrie Cassileth at the University of Pennsylvania Medical School, who had heard of Dr. Livingston's work and wished to investigate further, compared treatments given at that institution (consisting essentially of conventional approaches) with those provided at the Livingston Clinic. Cassileth demonstrated that both approaches provided *equal* benefits to patients in terms of improvement and cures, but that the Livingston approach was far better tolerated by the patients and had fewer side effects.

Ingrid's Story

Ingrid was a sixty-year-old woman from a small town just outside of Springfield, Missouri, who came to see me at the Livingston clinic for follow-up. She had been diagnosed as having metastatic ovarian cancer several years before, and after several rounds of chemotherapy, following surgery, she was still not well. Ingrid still had residual implants, which are nests of cancer cells that attach to the wall of the peritoneum, the lining of the abdominal and pelvic cavity. She had read about Dr. Livingston's work and made the trip to San Diego to receive the vaccines as well as the other immune-building materials and diet, along with large doses of intravenous vitamin C. After a two-week course of treatment and instruction, she went home with these materials and continued to use them for several years. When I saw her at the clinic, she was healthy but still not cured, as testing still showed the presence of cancerous ovarian cells.

I continued to treat Ingrid for several years in San Diego, and as luck would have it, I relocated my medical practice to Springfield, Missouri, where I continued to treat her for the next ten years. During that time she did quite well, except for her experiences with several courses of chemotherapy that reduced her white blood-cell count to the point that she became susceptible to pneumonia and had several life-threatening bouts with infection, until her immune system could regroup. With the use of the Livingston program and materials, although she was never cured, Ingrid kept her advanced cancer at bay for almost fifteen years! During most of that time, she was able to live a healthy, productive life with her family and community. Her gynecological oncologist, who followed her throughout that period, was initially opposed to her treatment at the Livingston Clinic, but over time was won over to its benefits. After several years he would reiterate to her the litany that we hear so often in this field: "I don't really understand what you are doing, but please keep it up. It's working." He often commented to her that his conventional treatment was clearly not responsible for her continued excellent state of health and her immune system's ability to keep the metastatic cancer at bay.

Ingrid's story is an excellent example of how an alternative approach, when combined with conventional treatment, produced many years of healthy living.

Alternative Approaches to Cancer Therapy

Are there other unique approaches that may be helpful for cancer patients? Yes, actually, too many to include here. While this is not intended to be a comprehensive discussion of the subject, I would like briefly to give a summary of some of those treatments that have the best track records and have been studied in the most detail. There are some general principles of alternative cancer therapy that many alternative clinics incorporate into their programs.

DIET

There is a great deal of well documented research showing that certain foods are good for our immune system, and other foods may be detrimental. The major points of agreement include the need to avoid sugar, preservatives, pesticides, and chemicals (translation: eating organic products, especially fresh fruits and vegetables and avoiding processed foods). Certain foods, such as broccoli, cauliflower, Brussels sprouts, and kale, contain phytonutrients, which have recently been shown to improve immune system functioning dramatically. Newer information about their preparation demonstrates that steaming them for one to two minutes is ideal for preserving the nutrients we wish to utilize. Dr. Patrick Quillin, who for many years has served as the nutritional director for Cancer Clinics of America, has written several excellent books on this subject.

SUPPLEMENTATION

The use of specific nutrients and supplements to improve the immune system is another component to most of these programs. These include high doses (25-50 g or 25,000 to 50,000 mg) of vitamin C given intravenously, along with selenium, zinc, vitamin A, Coenzyme Q10, and other anti-oxidants. You might wonder why the intravenous route of vitamin C is so essential, but there is significant disagreement about how much vitamin C the body can absorb when given orally. Several studies show that only 100 mg of vitamin C can be absorbed by the body when it is taken as often as every four hours, but other studies done by Dr. Linus Pauling show that much more can be absorbed. The bottom line is that regardless of how much vitamin C can be absorbed when taken orally, the intravenous use of vitamin C allows us to provide much more nutrient than we could ever get orally. Recent research by Dr. Mark Levine at the National Institute of Health has finally demonstrated how this works: the high doses of vitamin C given intravenously are converted in the extracellular tissues into high concentration of hydrogen peroxide, which can then attack the cancer cells.

VISUALIZATION TECHNIQUES

Originally proposed and researched by Drs. Carl and Stephanie Simonton and expanded by others, including Dr. Bernie Siegel, visualization techniques are another major component of most of these programs. Our knowledge of the tongue-twisting field of psychoneuroimmunology shows a clear relationship between our thoughts and feelings and the functioning of our immune system. Carl Simonton was a radiation oncologist who was able to prove that patients who could picture, or imagine, their immune systems killing off their cancers did far better clinically than those who did not make use of that faculty. Dozens of subsequent research papers have confirmed that observation. So, a positive outlook coupled with consistent visualization efforts aimed at visually improving the function of the immune system leads to much better outcomes. It is safe, costs nothing but a little time, and has no side effects. Dr. Livingston's program incorporated all of these elements into their treatments.

OTHER REMEDIES

Other programs and concepts which readers may wish to study include the following:
- *The Gerson Program* – named after a pioneering physician who first used high doses of vitamin C intravenously with extensive juicing, coffee enemas, and thyroid supplementation, among other interventions
- *Macrobiotic Diets* – as popularized by Michio Kushi, uses a fairly austere dietary program to mobilize immune system function
- *Herbal Treatments* – the Hoxsey treatment, mistletoe (Iscador)
- *Essiac tea, pau d'arco,* and *mushroom extracts* have been used by hundreds of patients with considerable success

- *The Burzynski Antineoplastons* – Dr. Burzynski isolated some unique peptides over thirty years ago, and has effectively used them in the treatment of a variety of cancers at his clinic in Houston, Texas
- *The Immuno-Augmentative Therapy program (IAP)* – introduced by Lawrence Burton in the Bahamas, uses again some unique peptides in cancer treatment .
- *Biologically Guided Chemotherapy* – introduced by Emanuel Revici, utilized a unique lipid chemistry approach to treatment
- *Laetrile*, so-called Vitamin B-17 – had some great success in the 1970s until the product was dramatically diluted by its manufacturer
- *Homeopathic Approaches* – including the Sanum remedies and Dr. Vincent Speckhart's electro-dermal screening remedies

These are but a few of the options available to those who are seeking other methods for healing. Several references in our bibliography can point the reader in these directions.

Alternative Approaches to Autoimmune Diseases

With other autoimmune diseases, too, the conventional approach is essentially suppressive but does not address the causes of autoimmunity. These diseases include rheumatoid arthritis, lupus erythematosus, Hashimoto's thyroiditis, multiple sclerosis, inflammatory bowel disease, and a host of other conditions, many of them less familiar to you. What brings about all of these conditions is an immune system which has become confused—it has started to attack its owner's tissue, mistakenly thinking it was attacking a foreign invader. For example, in rheumatoid arthritis, the immune system attacks the synovium, which is the membrane that lines the joints. When the synovium becomes inflamed, joint pain ensues, and that underlying inflammatory process may become generalized and affect other body tissues. In Hashimoto's thyroiditis, the thyroid gland is attacked, and eventually this process destroys all or part of the thyroid gland, creating a condition of hypothyroidism. In multiple sclerosis, it is the nerve tissue which is inflamed, causing a wide variety of nerve-related symptoms depending on the exact location of the affected tissues, involving, at times, the brain, spinal cord, or peripheral nerves.

For many years, our main therapy for these diseases was (and remains) high doses of cortisone in the form of prednisone. This may, in fact, be lifesaving and absolutely necessary for many patients. However, long-term use of prednisone is associated with a host of serious side effects, and will rarely cure the patient as it does not address the cause of the problem. There are many newer effective treatments, but they still put the patient at risk for life-threatening infections because they work by suppressing the immune system as a whole, not in a specific way.

On the other hand, there are a host of less toxic approaches that have had success with treating autoimmune diseases. We still do not adequately understand the causes of these conditions; hence, treatments are limited by our lack of knowledge. By looking at this wide variety of treatments, we may get a glimpse into what may underlie some of these diseases.

First I would like to refer back to our discussion of the Livingston vaccine. I described the original work that Dr. Livingston did on scleroderma, noting that the same bacterium that caused cancer also appeared to be involved in the development of autoimmune diseases. When she applied her vaccines to those conditions, she had a great deal of success.

I was able to go back into the files and come up with eighteen patients with scleroderma whom we had treated over a number of years. In fact, quite a few of the cases were active, so I was still following most of them. All were well documented diagnostically from university centers, so the diagnosis was not in question. Of the eighteen we treated with the Livingston vaccine, six were cured, six were markedly improved, and six showed no improvement—two-thirds of the patients responded positively to this treatment! You may not realize it, but conventional medicine is not capable of achieving these results. There is definite benefit of the use of these vaccines in autoimmune illness, and, when it works, it is clearly addressing the cause of that disease in that patient.

Recall also in the first chapter when I described the use of hypnosis and emotional release work in curing patients with rheumatoid arthritis and other autoimmune diseases: somehow, this process has the capacity to restore the immune system back into balance.

When we discussed mercury toxicity, I mentioned that this is often associated with autoimmune illness. I have personally seen several cases of rheumatoid arthritis and multiple sclerosis respond beautifully to the removal of mercury, and others have described this as well. What role does heavy metal toxicity play, therefore, in the weakening of the immune system, pushing it towards self-reactivity? Perhaps a very significant one.

We have also commented on the role of food allergy in autoimmunity. Many patients with rheumatoid arthritis and inflammatory bowel disease have responded well to or have even been cured by discovering the offending foods and removing them.

Perhaps in a similar way, in restoring balance to the bowel and removing toxins from the system, the practices of fasting, high colonics, and saunas have been used by naturopathic physicians for decades in the service of the successful treatment of these conditions.

More unusual treatments include bee venom therapy. Using controlled bee stings, or bee venom in different forms, has resulted in improvement in patients, particularly those with multiple sclerosis and rheumatoid arthritis. While some of you may be shaking your head at this one (I did, too, when I first encountered it), I have seen it work. The venom can be injected just under the skin (subcutaneously) over acupuncture points, or into areas of pain, particularly around joints, with great benefit.

Certain infections have been implicated in the development of autoimmunity, especially the HHV-6 virus and EBV virus, which we discussed earlier. Improvements have been noted, particularly in multiple sclerosis, by treatments directed at improving the immune system's ability to deal with those viruses, notably with the use of transfer factors.

Again, suggesting the possible involvement of bacterial infection in causing these diseases, Dr. Brown in Texas has published many papers showing the success of using low, long-term doses of tetracyclines (an antibiotic) in treating rheumatoid arthritis. I have personally seen similar results.

We have recently realized that vitamin D is deficient in the majority of our patients, and especially in those with autoimmune disease. By measuring and treating this deficiency, we are seeing great improvements in those patients. This will be discussed in more detail in the Afterword of this book.

Once you begin to investigate more deeply into these areas, you will find many other options for treatment, many of which are worthy of exploration. Hope abounds. Sometimes you have to take a creative step back to get a better perspective on the whole situation. This may help you to realize that no, you really haven't tried everything available in your search for a cure.

Further Reading

Cassileth, Barrie, et al. "Survival and Quality of Life among Patients Receiving Unproven as Compared with Conventional Cancer Therapy." *The New England Journal of Medicine* 324.17 (1991): 1180-1185.

Diamond, W. J., and W. L. Cowden. *Alternative Medicine Definitive Guide to Cancer.* Tiburon, CA: Future Medicine, 1997.

Livingston, Virginia. *Conquest of Cancer: Vaccines and Diet.* Waterside Products, New York: F. Watts, 1984.

Macomber, P. B. "Cancer and Cell Wall Deficient Bacteria." *Medical Hypotheses* 32 (1990): 1-9.

Quillin, Patrick. *Beating Cancer with Nutrition.* 4th ed. Carlsbad, CA: Nutrition Times, 2005.

Unconventional Cancer Treatments. Washington, D.C.: U.S. Congress Office of Technology Assessment, 1990.

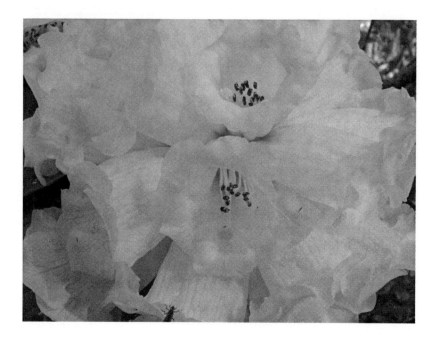

Chapter 22

Autism

How It All Fits Together

I've enjoyed creating mildly amusing chapter subtitles for this book, but somehow it doesn't feel right to do that with a chapter on autism. Having a good sense of humor is one thing, but there is absolutely nothing amusing about having a child who is struggling to function in every way.

My first contact with autistic children occurred when I went to medical school at the University of Chicago. During that sojourn, I had the opportunity to take some classes with Bruno Bettelheim, the medical researcher who ran the Autogenic School at the university. He was one of the first physicians to attempt a strategy to help these unfortunate autistic children. Back then, autism was extremely rare and was mostly thought to be a result of unusual genetic problems. Curing or improving autism in those days was always assumed to be a minor miracle.

Today, we have an epidemic of autism. In this country, 1 in 150 children is now diagnosed with autism, and in certain communities that incidence has increased to 1 in 50. And the form of autism has changed. Previously, children were abnormal from the start of their lives. They never developed properly, or walked or talked or made meaningful contact with their caregivers. What we are now seeing is primarily *regressive* autism. These children have normal births, grow and develop normally, talk and walk and cuddle, up until a certain point; then they take a sudden and dramatic backward turn and lose these abilities. Unfortunately, the conventional medical approach is to place these children on multiple medications to control their symptoms of out-of-control behaviors, tantrums, tics, "stimming" activities, and withdrawal from social contact.

As with many of the concepts presented in this book, "controlling" or "managing" symptoms can never result in a cure of an illness, as these treatments do not begin to address the cause. Most conventional physicians do not believe we have adequate knowledge of this cause and hence do not make any efforts to work with it. And once again, it is my belief, shared with an increasing number of physicians, that we have learned a great deal about this new and epidemic form of autism and can treat it by getting closer to the causes.

With autism, we have a very exciting story. The search for a cause began with Dr. Bernard Rimland's vision that a new approach was needed. In 1967, he founded the Autism Research Institute, which started by asking parents to rate the benefits of all of the treatments their children were receiving. The process was simple: parents scored each treatment as better, worse, or unchanged for every intervention they tried, including both conventional and alternative approaches. Over the course of time, a significant number of observations accumulated. Using a scale of one as meaning "unchanged," less than one as meaning "worse," and more than one as "better," it was clear that some medications were, if anything, mildly helpful. But a host of natural treatments clearly made much bigger differences. It was noted that digestive changes, including removing milk and wheat from the diet and looking for food allergies, made big differences and were highly rated by parents. In addition, by treating occult intestinal yeast and bacterial infections; removing toxins from the system, especially mercury and lead; treating methylation defects; and supplementing with vitamins and nutrients, patients showed a marked improvement. Some children were cured, and most got better. Does this whole process sound familiar? It should, since we've devoted whole chapters of this book to all of these interventions and concepts.

Looking at this bigger picture, more researchers became intrigued with the possibility of helping these children. Some of the most passionate, of course, began their journey when their own children were diagnosed with autism. When your own child is affected, this is powerful motivation to find answers. In 1995, this body of information evolved into the Defeat Autism Now! movement, which continues to integrate new information and research into the treatment program, and is taught to more and more physicians as time moves on. As parents learned about the epidemic, their need to have these treatments available and supervised by knowledgeable physicians led to this whole biomedical approach, and large medical conferences are held several times a year to facilitate this exchange of information.

What we have learned thus far is that the key areas of imbalance in these children are their brain chemistry (no surprise) and their guts. The latter shouldn't be much of a surprise, either, to readers of this book, when we reflect that the gut contains more neurotransmitters than the brain and is often referred to as the "little brain." The gut is also associated with the immune system, 60 percent of which is present in the gut as the *Gut-Associated Lymphoid Tissue* (GALT). Although the neurological effects of autism are in many ways more obvious, the intestinal symptoms have long been present but mostly overlooked. During recent autism conferences, gastroenterologist after gastroenterologist has presented material on the marked prevalence of every type of intestinal diagnosis in autistic children. The autism groups have discovered that treating this condition starts with "normalizing" gut function.

The key imbalances, which we've seen in other chronic conditions, are food allergies, especially sensitivity to casein (milk protein) and gluten (wheat protein). One major starting point for treatment is to take autistic children off of each of these separately, followed if necessary with more elaborate tests for other food allergies. If an autistic child improves with simple elimination of food allergies, we're off to a good start. Another starting point closely linked with food sensitivities is looking for and treating chronic yeast (*Candida*) and bacterial infections. Sixty to 70 percent of regressive autistic children respond well to these interventions. We then shift our attention to toxicities: evaluating these children for the presence of heavy metals, especially mercury and lead, and chemicals and pesticides, which are so prevalent in our environment. New studies also show a clear relationship between exposure to pesticides in agricultural settings and the incidence of autism.

Studies also suggest a relationship between vaccine usage and autism in several ways. First, until recently, many childhood vaccines had significant amounts of thimerosol, a mercury-containing preservative. When vaccines were "bundled," or given in large batches at the same time, doctors were inadvertently injecting large amounts of mercury into these children's systems. The developing nervous system of a young child is especially vulnerable to these toxins. While this situation has improved somewhat, thimerosol is still present in appreciable amounts in the flu vaccine, which is now recommended for most children. Second, and separately, there is reason to suspect that the measles vaccine (*Rubeola*, or the R in MMR vaccine), as a live virus vaccine, may actually cause infection in some cases. Although the virus used in this vaccine is supposed to be "attenuated," or weakened and benign, it would appear that it is not always so, and the ensuing infection may trigger autism in susceptible children. *Susceptible* is the operative word here.

We have gathered enough information now that a model for the evaluation and treatment of regressive autism has been proposed by the Autism Research Institute group. We have also begun to learn more about the details of genetic predisposition, which we can now measure by simple blood tests. These genetic predispositions, coupled with a variety of exposures to heavy metal and chemical and mold toxins, may well explain how regressive autism develops, and also provide a rationale for treatment. Some of these exposures include the exposure of a susceptible child to multiple rounds of antibiotic, which trigger intestinal dysbiosis, and then set off the development of food allergy. Toxic exposures may additionally weaken or deplete the all-important methylation pathway so that these unfortunate children cannot produce the natural materials that are required for healing.

Jill James at the University of Arkansas has completed some meticulous research that provides evidence for these methylation deficiencies and also demonstrates clinical response to a simple supplement-replacement pathway. James has taken this one step further by showing deficiencies on the part of the parents of these children, and she is currently engaged in a more extensive research effort to both study and treat these imbalances.

As heartbreaking as the diagnosis of autism is for all parents, this model provides real hope for them and gives us impetus to embrace this new model of understanding and treatment.

Isaac's Story

Isaac was a five-year-old whom I initially saw in May 2007 at his mother's request. She had seen two medical specialists who had made the diagnosis of Asperger's syndrome, which is currently considered a variety of autism. Isaac had developed normally up until about two years of age, when his behavior began to change. His mother felt that these changes seemed to occur following vaccinations he received at that time. His mother observed that Isaac would often go into his own little world. He was having increasing difficulty making social contact with others, especially if they were not family or well known to him. When people would get too close, Isaac would literally tell them to back off, or he would shy away. It was difficult to get him to leave the house without taking a host of toys with him to keep him entertained. He appeared to be quite intelligent (common with Asperger's children) but his speech was "off" at times, and he was not yet toilet trained.

When we tested Isaac's stool, he had overgrowth of the yeast Candida Albicans as well as the toxic bacteria Klebsiella and Enterobacter. We initially treated him with Nystatin and Diflucan, and prescribed the use of melatonin for difficulties with sleep, which is commonly seen in autistic children. The use of the methylation protocol made a big difference in Isaac's behaviors from the moment we started, although initially there was a slight increase in his tic behaviors, and some social withdrawal, which rapidly improved. As he was a big milk drinker, we eliminated the consumption of milk to see if this would help. It made little difference.

He was placed in a special educational program at school, and within a few months of beginning our treatment, Isaac was completely potty trained and was able to ride the bus to school by himself. At this point his mother felt he was 40 percent better than when we'd started. When we retested his stool in March 2008, he had several bacterial pathogens and two species of Candida on culture. At that time, he'd gone off the methylation protocol and was encouraged to resume it, which he did. We treated the intestinal overgrowth with Nizoral, uva ursi, and undecylenic acid, and he improved markedly. By the end of summer school, July 2008, he was ready to resume regular classes with just a small amount of time out of his school day (twenty-five minutes) devoted to special training in speech and motor skills. He was able to interact much better with his peers and no longer exhibited the anxiety and tics he had prior to treatment. His mother was thrilled with his progress.

Unfortunately, just prior to the start of school, Isaac was given four bundled immunizations, including the MMR vaccine. His mother had been concerned about his possible reactions to those immunizations, but Isaac's pediatrician was insistent. Within twenty-four hours of the shots, his mother reported, "I've never seen him so nervous or jumpy." Over that first week, his regression continued as he became increasingly fearful, and began holding back his willingness to interact with others. One week after the immunizations he broke out in a finely grained, red rash all over his body. We were moving back to square one.

Thankfully, with resumption of his supplements and treatment program, and a little time, this exacerbation resolved within a few weeks and Isaac resumed his school activities successfully; his gains in behavioral function returned, and he has continued to make steady progress.

Nina's Story

In January 2008, I had my first visit with a very delightful seven-year-old named Nina. She had been diagnosed with petit mal ("absence") seizures at the age of three, and over time had been found to have difficulties with focus and attention and sleep. She was closely followed by a pediatric neurologist who diagnosed her with ADHD, which many experts consider part of the autism spectrum. He placed her on the medication Concerta, which seemed to help initially. After eighteen months, Nina's mother had begun to wonder whether the side effects of Concerta were outweighing its benefits. Nina had also been placed on Lamactical, an anti-seizure medication, but EEGs (brain wave testing) continued to be abnormal, and she had frequent headaches, averaging three times per week. The family did quite a bit of research over the internet, as is common in my practice, and they were hoping that some of these newer concepts could be helpful for their young girl.

At our first visit, after collecting the appropriate information, I began with some osteopathic cranial manipulation. When she returned, six weeks later, headaches were markedly diminished. We added vitamin B6 and the supplement L-taurine to her program. We started the process of looking for food allergies and possible heavy metal toxicity. On a DMSA challenge test, moderate amounts of nickel, lead, and mercury were discovered, and she was started on DMSA twice weekly. One mg of melatonin was added at bedtime.

By the next visit, Nina's sleep had improved, headaches were rare, and she had experienced only one significant seizure. Her mother told me that Nina was substantially better already. We added the methylation supplement protocol, and continued her cranial manipulation. By July, her mother reported to us that Nina was "happier and more energetic." She was no longer having any seizure activity, and headaches were few and far between. She had been tutored that summer and had caught up to her grade level for educational instruction. Her mother was able to say that her concentration and focus had improved dramatically. Off medication completely, Nina no longer exhibited symptoms of ADHD and was free from seizures.

You can see how combining a nutritional approach with osteopathic manipulation, removing toxins, and providing methylation support was able to produce marked improvement in just six months. Restoring health and improved brain function for these children is clearly possible.

I am in awe of the effort and dedication of the parents of these autistic children. Their willingness to step out of conventional boundaries to find the help their children need is inspiring. They will not accept "you'll just have to learn to live with this" as an answer, and through their efforts, we are pushed to dig ever deeper for answers and solutions. The good news is that this intense search is often rewarded with the evolution of a healthier, happier child and a grateful family.

Further Reading

Baker, Sidney, and Jon Pangborn. *Autism: Effective Biomedical Treatments (Have We Done Everything We Can For This Child? Individuality In An Epidemic)*. 2nd ed. San Diego: Autism Research Institute, 2005.

McCandless, Jaquelyn. *Children with Starving Brains: A Medical Treatment Guide for Autism Spectrum Disorder*. 4th ed. Putney, VT: Bramble Books, 2009.

McCarthy, Jenny. *Louder Than Words: A Mother's Journey in Healing Autism*. New York: Dutton, 2007.

The Bigger Picture:
A Look toward the Future

With all of this new information available for study, I would like to complete this book by putting this all into perspective. Thus far much of this book has been directed to the evolving understanding of how body chemistry becomes disordered and can be repaired. Now I'd like to step back a little and look at the bigger picture.

The first area for us to explore is an important one: why have so many individuals become ill in such a short period of time? Despite all of the advances of modern medicine, why are cancer and autoimmune disease and fibromyalgia and chronic fatigue and autism and Alzheimer's disease continuing to become more prevalent at an alarming rate? Many scientists have studied this critical question, and to many of us it appears that what has changed is our environment. Chapter 23 explores how this has happened and attempts to clarify this frightening phenomenon.

Next, I will explore the importance of *listening*. This includes the need for me to listen really carefully to what my patients are expressing, so that I can begin the diagnostic process. It also includes patients' needs to listen to their bodies so that they can act accordingly. Chapter 24 delves into this vital but often overlooked area.

The next chapter is an unusual one, in that it will delve into the seldom discussed relationship between money and healing. Chapter

25 looks at the important interactions between patients and healthcare providers as decisions are made about how to spend money in the service of health.

Chapter 26 will explore the spiritual dimensions of health and healing. Our attitudes toward our illness, our bodies, and our families play an important role in determining how we will fare. We must courageously explore this to prevent anything from limiting the natural healing processes.

In Chapter 27 I will present a brief story about the power of caring.

Chapter 23

Ecotoxicity: How Our Environment Is Making You Sick

Only the Tip of the Iceberg

aving gotten this far, an obvious question finally emerges: "Why is all of this biochemical mayhem happening now?" There must be reasons for the emergence of this epidemic of fibromyalgia, chronic fatigue, autism, ADHD, asthma, cancer, Alzheimer's, and Parkinson's disease. I believe there are, but none at this moment are scientifically confirmed or proven. Despite the lack of proof, I can't help but speculate on what might be going on here. I and many other physicians and scientists suspect that there are chemical, energetic, emotional, and spiritual components involved.

For starters, we seem to have lost touch with what makes us human. As a species relatively new to this planet, we seem to think we can create a world separate from the one we are actually living in. For most of our time on earth, we have lived in some degree of harmony with nature: we hunted, we farmed, we gathered, we fished. We have always had to pay careful attention to the natural world in order to live in harmony with nature to survive. If we hunted- or fished-out a species of game, we had to leave that area and move on, so we learned not to do so. If we didn't treat the soil properly, we learned that it would not produce in abundance.

But now we've rather suddenly lost our intimate contact with the natural world. The most glaring example of this is the insidious proliferation of technology in our lives. It seems like you just can't go anywhere these days without being deluged by media. It is a rare restaurant that doesn't have multiple television sets visible or audible from every seat in the room. When and how did this happen? I am especially aware of this when I am in airports, noticing that they are filled with people on cell phones, talking in raised voices, oblivious to the world around them. This forces all of those in their vicinity (in this instance, me) to respond in some way to this outpouring of sound energy. I can try to tune it out, become irritated, listen in with interest, or wear blocking earphones to deal with it. But deal with it I must, because I can't just ignore it. Perversely, this distances me from my own perceptions and my own life and intrudes upon my physiology in a most unhealthy way. And people seem to take this for granted to the point that they are oblivious to what is happening around them.

I take a walk with my family in a natural setting, and almost every jogger, bicyclist, or fellow walker is wearing earphones and is plugged in to a virtual world which separates them from the world in which they are moving. This is a deeply spiritual problem. For many of us, one of the simplest ways to be close to our god is through a natural setting: a sunrise, sunset, blue sky with fleecy clouds, stream running through a grove of trees, or a field of flowers. But if we're not present to it—if we stay constantly and remotely connected to these virtual worlds—we no longer take the time to see, hear, smell, or feel our real world. So we have the bizarre experience of being in it, but not really taking part in it. And as this strange dissociation from the world we inhabit continues, we have an increasingly strained relationship with the natural world. We're now seeing the effects of global warming, the obliteration of rain forests, the building of huge tracts of housing on good farmland, and the use of untested chemicals on our soils and in our homes and schools. Why should any of this come as such a surprise? No one seems to be paying much attention to the bigger picture.

We've become numb. So numb that our media resorts to gorier pictures and more intense, fear-based news and images to get our attention. So numb that even the most realistic movies barely move our audiences. I read studies that show that an extraordinary percentage of Americans are currently taking antidepressants, and from a glance at my patient population, I believe them. Basically, antidepressants numb us up. So how, in this numb, stressed, out-of-touch universe that we are creating, can we even notice how we feel? It's simple—we can't. Our bodies were designed to notice imbalances and bring them to our attention so that we could fix them. If we can't do that because we're numb, we can get really sick before we realize we need to do something about it. When we do come to our senses, we often find that our medical providers have no idea how to address these profound biological imbalances in any sort of practical way, so they tell us we are stressed and it's "in our heads." All they can do is suggest we go elsewhere for treatment. And what will they give us for treatment? Why, more antidepressants of course!

Where can we go for help? Where must we look in order to address this problem?

We have to go home, and by home I mean back into our own bodies, our own lives—to recover ourselves. It's not outside of us; it's inside. And we've lost the awareness of both what we need to do and how to do it. That means we need to change our relationship with technology. I am not suggesting that technology is malevolent or that it has no place in our modern world. I am saying that our relationship to it is way out of balance, and most important, we need to be *aware* of that relationship so that we don't completely lose contact with the natural world. But how can we do that? Many of my patients work in front of computer screens all day long and come home to more of the same. We pay bills with it, buy airline tickets with it, "surf" it, communicate with it, are beguiled by it. It's not just going to go away, nor should it.

So we clearly need a new relationship with technology. How, exactly, can we do this? I am not going to propose glib answers to a very difficult problem, but I can say that the essence of this problem lies in the loss of our abilities to notice our own thoughts, our own feelings, our own perceptions, when we are deluged with electronic stimuli all around us. We must find some personal way to slow the deluge for long enough that we can recover ourselves, and not allow ourselves to be swept up into it. I believe we can do this.

❖

Pesticides and Chemicals

Another major need for our awareness comes from the following:

> For the first time in the history of the world, every human being is now subjected to contact with dangerous chemicals, from the moment of conception until death. In the less than two decades of their use, the synthetic pesticides have been so thoroughly distributed throughout the animate and inanimate world that they occur virtually everywhere . . . . To adjust to these chemicals would require time on the scale that is nature's; it would require not merely the years of a man's life but the life of generations. (Carson 7, 15)

It may come as a shock to learn that these are not newly-penned sentences, but were written in 1962 by Rachel Carson in her groundbreaking book, *Silent Spring*. The two decades referred to are now six. Although the publishing of her book led to the prohibition of the pesticide DDT, a recent study shows that even forty years since DDT has been banned from our environment, fat biopsies show that virtually all of us still have DDT in our bodies!

The chemical industry releases approximately 500 new chemicals every year. It is estimated that there are perhaps 80,000 chemicals in our environment, and only 500 of them have been adequately studied in terms of their effects on humans. What is worse, there are virtually no studies of how those chemicals interact with each other. We are swimming in a sea of chemicals that are almost certainly poisoning our bodies, our whole world, and we are not allowing ourselves to measure the effects that this has upon us. This should be a terrifying fact, but most of us go along blithely with an indifferent attitude: "If they were dangerous, surely we'd know by now." But remember, it took many years for us to discover that DDT had profound effects on the environment and our hormones, and needed to be banned.

We have evidence now, that many plastics and common chemicals in our environment are xenoestrogens, *xeno* signifying "foreign." What this means is that these unnatural chemicals are so close in their biochemical structure to our natural hormones (estrogen being the one named here) that they *behave* like hormones in our bodies, not only confusing our chemistry, but making it nearly impossible to eliminate or detoxify them because they are not natural. We have discovered that many of these chemicals, even in exquisitely small amounts, block and interfere with our normal hormonal function. There is solid evidence that male sperm counts and fertility rates globally have decreased by over 50 percent in the past twenty years! Do we not think this is really significant? No, we gloss over it, hoping that magically, like the epidemics of illness we are currently seeing, it will just go away. We rarely drink the water available to us from our taps anymore. We drink from plastic bottles, thinking that this water is purer; but is it? We have reasons to doubt. Study after study shows us that exposure to every type of plastic in our environment has the potential to leach chemical toxins into our bodies. What *is* safe? I no longer know the answer to that question, but I do know that we must find out, and soon.

I and many others believe that it is our polluted world that is making us so sick. Some of us are more sensitive than others, and they are the ones who are coming in to my office now. I don't think it will be very long before these numbers increase dramatically. Those who have felt immune will somehow have to deal with these environmental toxins, too. This means *polluted* not only in terms of chemicals, but also pollutions of noise, electromagnetic radiation, information, and stressors, amongst others. This is sensory stimulation overload, with which we are ill-equipped to cope, yet we rarely even acknowledge. For example, as I write these words on my word processor, I am aware that after about two hours in front of this screen, I can no longer think clearly. Unless I allow my awareness of this to become conscious, I will continue to plug along until I can no longer write coherently. If I can then go outside or take a walk, this will fade after thirty minutes to an hour. Discussions with hundreds of patients over the past few years have convinced me that my experience is not unique.

Some of my patients are much more sensitive to electromagnetic effects and are rendered almost non-functional with everyday exposures. The proliferation of radio towers and beacons in our world has gone almost unnoticed, but that does not mean that they do not affect us. When I worked with Dr. Norman Shealy a dozen years ago, by carefully monitoring the brain waves of sensitive patients, we were able to clearly demonstrate that in the presence of electromagnetic radiation (a simple clock, for example), those patients would move from functional alpha and beta brainwave patterns into random delta brain wave patterns that correlated precisely with their loss of cognitive function.

Until now, most people have taken an "I'm O.K., so what's *your* problem?" approach to this. The implication here is that an innate sensitivity to chemicals, electromagnetic radiation, or foods must be somehow psychological rather than a physical, non-controllable reaction. When viewed with a little more compassion, some people respond, "There but for the grace of God go I." Neither of these attitudes reflects a realistic compassion or understanding of the problem. Sorry, but we're all an integral part of this universe. There is no rug to sweep this under. It will not go away.

It is like there is an elephant in the room, and we have all agreed not to notice it or talk about it. Remember our discussion on cognitive dissonance? Here is another example. You see, the elephant *is* in the room, and denying its existence will not make it go away. There are obviously tremendous economic pressures to avoid this discussion, but I am convinced that our lives will depend on our immediate admission of this huge problem and not delaying one more minute to deal with it. I don't see that we have any choice.

If we're going to talk about health, we have to include the bigger picture in this discussion, and this is just the tip of the iceberg.

Further Reading

Carson, Rachel. *Silent Spring*. New York: Houghton Mifflin, 1962.

Colborn, Theo, Dianne Dumanoski, and John P. Meyers. *Our Stolen Future: Are We Threatening Our Fertility, Intelligence, and Survival?—A Scientific Detective Story*. New York: Plume, 1997.

Krimsky, Sheldon, and Lynn Goldman. *Hormonal Chaos: The Scientific and Social Origins of the Environmental Endocrine Hypothesis*. Baltimore: The Johns Hopkins UP, 2002.

Chapter 24

Understanding Complexity in Human Beings

Friends, Americans, Countrymen: Lend Me Your Ears

*I*t is difficult for me to explain to others the process we use to help people regain their health. I think the reason for this is, in essence, that it is too simple and does not fit into the model used by medical practice today. That model, as we've discussed, includes a very brief interview with the patient, followed by lots of high-tech testing and prescription writing. It seems pretty obvious that this model has no real chance of working or being effective, since it eliminates the possibility of allowing the patient to tell her story and express her feelings—there's simply no time for it.

In my opinion, the essence of helping people boils down to intense listening, remaining ever attentive to their descriptions of their personal health. While listening to patients should obviously be the most important part of our medical interaction, I throw in the word *intense* to emphasize that this is not merely sitting in the same room with patients, but reflects the hard work of really paying attention to them as they speak. This means attending not only to their words, but also to the pauses between words, the words that are emphasized (hence more emotionally charged and meaningful), as well as their body language and facial expressions as they relate their stories (leaning forward in the chair, legs abruptly crossed, sudden deep breaths, sighing, eye contact or lack thereof). In short, I must take in the totality of that individual human being and allow the totality of my being to get involved so that it registers information about what is really important to that individual, as he relates his stories. Somewhere in that entire presentation are the clues we need to be of help. If the physician is busy working at her computer, keying in the patient's information, or pressed for time, wondering how she can possibly fit into the morning schedule the required "output" of "productivity," it is clear that meaningful listening cannot take place. Somewhere in the past fifteen to twenty years, we went from being physicians to becoming "providers," and that seemingly simple linguistic change has had a profound impact on the practice of medicine.

The closest model that approximates a process of deep listening may be found in the field of osteopathic medicine, which we discussed in Chapter 17. This may come as a surprise to some who aren't aware of the osteopathic profession or how it differs from that of conventional medicine. There is, in fact, a deep philosophical underpinning to osteopathy, which is surprisingly absent from that of allopathic medicine. There are four basic principles of osteopathy, as outlined by Rollin Becker, D.O., in his book, *Life in Motion*:

1. The body is a unit.
2. The body possesses self-regulatory mechanisms.
3. Structure and function are reciprocally interrelated.
4. Rational therapy is based upon an understanding of the body's self regulatory mechanism and the body's interrelationship of structure and function.

The steps taken to address healing the body are based on these principles:

1. Accept the Living Mechanism in you and the patient.
    Life is always trying to express health.
2. Surrender comes after acceptance.
    Accept the fact that what the mechanism is telling you is true.
3. Develop palpatory skills.
    The body is smarter than you are, so learn to learn from it.

A great deal of wisdom is buried in these succinct comments. What Dr. Becker is driving at is at the heart of our interaction with our patients: we need to change our thinking that our job is to fix what is wrong with the patient. Rather, we must find a way to understand that there is a deep core of health in these patients already (after all, here they are in front of you, fully alive). This understanding needs to be accessed by both doctor and patient in order to harness the forces of healing. The key word here is *accessed*. This means listening, sensing, feeling, and paying attention, so that we can reach the patient's own self-healing mechanisms and begin to move forward.

The beauty and brilliance of this concept is that it recognizes that patients essentially heal themselves; we don't do the healing for them. Missing the truth of this is what has gotten the field of medicine moving down the wrong path in its approach to evaluating and treating chronic illness. In the current philosophy of conventional medicine, both physicians and patients are under the misperception that the physician is doing the healing. So, the patient turns over the responsibility for healing to the physician, and the physician accepts it. If both accept this unwritten contract, they are in trouble. The patients are abnegating their own responsibilities here, and the doctor is taking on responsibilities that are literally impossible to fulfill. This is a recipe for disaster.

Let's take a simple example. If a patient comes to me with pneumonia, and I give him a prescription for antibiotics, he assumes I've done my job. He thinks the antibiotic prescription will heal him. And if he gets better, he will assume that I and/or the antibiotic have cured him. But no antibiotic is capable of wiping out every bacterial cell in the body. The antibiotic allows the patient's immune system to get a leg up, a good head start on the process. But the total eradication of the bacterial or viral invaders is completely dependent on the ability of that patient's immune system to finish the job and mop up. If it can't do that, the infection will continue to smolder and the patient will stay sick.

Healing, therefore, depends almost entirely on the patient's own immune system and not on the antibiotic. I suspect that both patients and physicians have forgotten this, which leads to the odd interactions that now occur between them. If the patient isn't getting well after being given an antibiotic, the doctor feels responsible: "Maybe I used the wrong medication, or maybe I didn't prescribe it for long enough, or maybe I've got the wrong diagnosis, or maybe. . . . " To make things worse, the patient comes to believe that the doctor is responsible and returns to the office worried and upset. But what's really happened here is that we've missed the point. The doctor and patient need to work together to harness the patient's healing powers and find some way to stimulate that immune system to work properly.

Perhaps the patient I mentioned earlier contracted pneumonia because he was stressed or exhausted from working long hours or dealing with a family emergency. Perhaps the structure of his rib cage and his ability to ventilate properly were compromised by a seemingly insignificant fall, last week, when she caught herself awkwardly by her arms as she fell. Perhaps his immune system was weakened by his diet (for several weeks he had consumed almost nothing but fast food eaten on the run). All of this may need to be addressed before true healing can take place. But if both physician and patient believe that a different antibiotic should be prescribed (in the seven minutes allotted to this visit) and that this will fix the problem, there is the distinct possibility that both are likely to be mistaken and that healing will be delayed even more. The patient may then get even more ill and even more frustrated with the lack of progress from this medical interaction.

Returning to the principles of osteopathy expressed by Dr. Becker: from the beginning of our interaction, we should be searching for the sources of health that the patient brings to the table, and harness those to move forward. What exactly might this mean? Well, it could mean discussing the patient's current stressors and ways to cope better, from the outset. It could mean discussing the effects of smoking tobacco and drinking alcohol. It could mean discussing diet and its effect on the immune system: sugar consumption and fast foods are known to weaken the immune system, so if you are treating your pneumonia and eat most of your meals at McDonald's, this might well influence your ability to heal. It could mean discussing the use of herbs and supplements that are known to improve immune functioning, such as vitamin C, Echinacea, goldenseal, or colloidal silver for an acute viral infection. It could mean exploring the patient's physical structure more carefully. Does the patient have any restrictions to movement of his or her rib cage or diaphragm (caused by an old fall, or tension perennially held in the chest) that could be treated manually, which would allow better ventilation of the lungs and speed healing (or prevent recurrence).

Searching for those sources of health could also mean looking at the patient's thinking process and emotional response to pneumonia: "I always get sick every winter and it goes to my lungs and it takes months to go away" is a common expression. This predisposes that individual to get sick because she believes she will get sick every winter, which opens the door to the very event she fears by direct effects of her beliefs and thoughts upon the immune system. The mind exerts a powerful effect on the body that is not always beneficial, unless it is recognized and harnessed properly.

You can see that doing this sort of analysis cannot easily be limited to a seven-minute visit. Clearly, it would not only take more time, but it also presents a completely different approach to how we provide medical care. This model is more comprehensive, more logical and inclusive, and more likely to produce the desired results. It also changes the relationship or interaction between the doctor and the patient, so we are working together and we each have a responsibility for the outcome.

This is not a new paradigm. It has been around for centuries and was beautifully expressed in the osteopathic principles quoted above. Unfortunately, it has been neglected, and we are all the worse for it. The more complicated and long-standing a patient's suffering, the more difficult it is for us to understand it and to find some way to recognize, encourage, and stimulate the patient's own healing abilities to come forth. For some individuals, this information is so deeply buried, that this process is going to take a lot of time. However, the clues will only emerge through careful listening and visits to the drawing board over and over again.

Calvin's Story

I had been treating sixty-two-year-old Calvin for several years. Initially he had only needed some osteopathic manipulation for recurrent neck and shoulder pain, and I was able to help him with that over the course of several months. Several years later, he developed the onset of intense chest pain, and we referred him to a cardiologist who was able to help him heal without difficulty.

However, for the past two years, Calvin had been complaining of vague muscle aches and cramping, along with the insidious onset of difficulty with focus and concentration and headaches. Since Calvin was an attorney, this was more than a mere nuisance; it was interfering with his work. He had also gotten a bit depressed, which we presumed came from some serious stressors in his life, and we placed him on a small dose of antidepressant medication. After consultation with other physicians, he began to suspect that he had had adult onset attention-deficit difficulties for many years, and we added the use of Adderall, a stimulant, to help with his mental functioning. The medication appeared to be working, and he basically seemed content with our treatment. But six months ago he came into the office with a new complaint: he had developed paresthesias (sensations of numbness and tingling) down both arms and legs, in patterns that did not reflect the usual nerve distributions.

This new symptom produced that "aha" moment, when suddenly information falls into place and makes sense. I asked Calvin about whether he had noticed any mold in his home. I was not surprised when he related that he had smelled a lot of "mustiness" over what appeared to be the open beams of his home, and there had been some water leakage from his furnace several years ago, as well. When his home was carefully inspected, he did indeed have mold over many areas of his home, and most worrisome, in the heating and cooling systems.

We treated the mold toxicity (see Chapter 11) with Questran and Actos, and within two weeks Cal's paresthesias had virtually disappeared, along with the headaches. He reported marked improvement in his muscle spasms and cramps that had bothered him for several years. His depression had lifted, and the focus and concentration issues had significantly improved, so that he no longer required his stimulant or antidepressant medication.

He still needed to proceed with the remediation of his home, and he did have mild to moderate exacerbations of his symptoms each time he was additionally exposed to mold in other settings. But the mystery of his illness had been resolved.

❖

This story illustrates how important it is that each practitioner (in this case, myself) continues to keep his mind and ears open so that new information will be able to be received and processed properly. In this case, one new symptomatic detail allowed all of the previous data to fall into a clear and understandable pattern. Now we had something to work with, and now we could move toward healing. As I continue to reiterate, without a clear diagnosis, it is awfully difficult to achieve healing. And it is only by listening, carefully and whole-heartedly, that we can obtain the clues we need to make that diagnosis.

Further Reading

Brooks, Rachel, ed. *Life in Motion: The Osteopathic Vision of Rollin E. Becker, D.O.* Portland, OR: Stillness, 2001.

Sutherland, Adah S., and Anne Wales, eds. *Contributions of Thought: The Collected Writings of William Garner Sutherland, D.O.* 2nd ed. Fort Worth, TX: Sutherland Cranial Teaching Foundation, 1998.

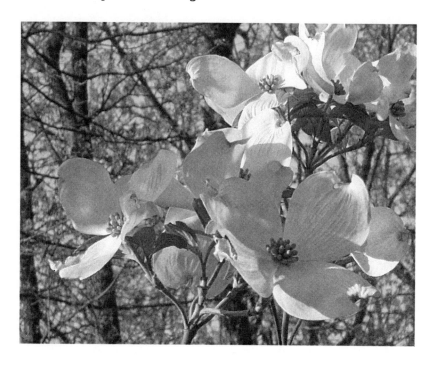

Chapter 25

The Pursuit of Healing

Does It Really Cost an Arm and a Leg?

*N*ow we come to a very difficult subject: the interaction between finances, attitudes, and healing.

Sometimes, money does matter. But it's more complicated than that. If you had a severe, debilitating illness that interfered with all aspects of your life, how much would you pay to correct it? As a physician with his sights set on healing (since this is the world I inhabit every day), to me, all people should be willing to move heaven and earth to regain their health. From my perspective, biased as it is, there is not much that is more important than your health. However, I have also learned that health and healing are not everyone else's highest goal or value. So I have to modify my goals (after all, it is your health-care visit) to make them jibe with those of my patients.

Patients will endlessly surprise me. Some of my wealthier patients will not spend a dime more than their insurance coverage will allow on their health. They will not authorize testing or use supplements or medications, and some of them will even say, "If my insurance company won't cover it, I must not need it." I am not aware of the enlightened philosophical nature of insurance companies, nor of their intense desire to be helpful at all times. Rather, it has seemed to me that they will do everything conceivable to deny claims whenever possible. On the other hand, many of my poorer patients will do everything they can to pay for every test I suggest, and take to heart every recommendation I make. Can you guess which of these patients do the best?

In a way, patients' attitudes toward the costs of medical care are like a Rorschach test, or barometer, of the kind of progress they'll make. Those who, from the beginning, tell me, "Do what it takes, I just want to get better," almost invariably do so. Those who "nickel and dime" me from the first visit, asking, "Which of those tests are the cheapest, which ones can I put off?" are likely to have a halting, up-and-down process, with excruciatingly slow to little improvement.

While some of this is about money, much more is about attitude. A genuine, whole-hearted desire to get well is required for a successful journey. Rarely does it work when a patient is not committed to the effort involved. And it's not just about money; it is also about the commitment of time and effort. Making dietary changes, taking supplements and medications at the correct times, learning relaxation techniques and really looking into one's attitudes towards healing or changing the stressful impediments of one's life takes a great deal of effort and discipline. Without that discipline, healing may not occur. I don't just sit down and write a prescription or hand you a supplement, and then you simply heal. Usually, once chronic illness has set in, quite a bit more effort is necessary.

When patients don't care to know about the financial aspects of our interactions, or if they have no financial responsibility for that interaction (with Medicaid or Medicare patients, for example), it profoundly impacts our interaction. Since our current medical system is largely based around these systems, we have lost the awareness of how important this is to the healing process. If people are not personally involved in the process of paying for the services they receive, they are distanced from our interaction and this diminishes their responsibility for their part of our interaction. It is not the amount of money that is exchanged that matters. I am simply stating that the actual interchange of money between us, no matter how small, adds immeasurably to our interaction. When that doesn't happen, it lessens our relationship.

One example of this would be how Medicare patients respond to the financial aspects of our relationship. When a patient pays me directly for my services, we have an immediate connection. They become a part of their healing. When they don't pay me directly, and the payment is from out there somewhere, they are much less involved in this process. For many years, I did not accept Assignment from Medicare. That simply means that those patients paid me directly on the day they saw me, and Medicare reimbursed them several weeks later. When we switched to accepting Assignment, it meant that the patient did not pay me at the time of service, and we were reimbursed later by Medicare. You might think that there was not much difference in those scenarios, but actually, yes, there was. When patients paid me, they did much better. They were much more committed to their healing and took a more active part in everything we outlined. When they no longer paid me, that commitment significantly decreased, and those patients shifted into an "if Medicare doesn't cover it, I must not need it" framework. They were much less likely to take an active part in their own care. They increasingly declined testing or procedures which weren't completely covered by Medicare. Consequently, their progress dropped off significantly.

Unfortunately, many useful tests, critical to diagnosis and treatment, are not covered by insurance (see examples throughout this book), and without them, we are working with our hands tied behind our backs. Without an understanding of and commitment to the cost of medical procedures, we are trying to swim upstream. How willing patients are to shoulder some of these costs is a clear statement of their commitment to healing. Those patients who wrestle with me over the cost of each and every test definitely do not fare as well. Their lack of commitment to healing is readily seen in this arena and reflects predictably on the treatment outcomes.

When a patient presents with a desire for disability, often the patient does not understand that this is antithetical to the healing process. It is not possible to seek both healing and financial gain simultaneously. Psychologically, when patients determine that they are entitled to disability, the vast majority cannot do so in good faith without unconsciously taking on the role of suffering, forever, in order to earn it. Alas, I cannot recall a single patient on or seeking disability who was able to fully heal. Often, as such patients make progress, they get to the point where they are almost well, and then they invariably have a serious setback that puts us back to square one. It is almost as if psychologically they cannot give up their disability, even for health. Now, for some, the reason may be financial, fearing loss of income and not knowing if they can return to the work force, even if they are well. For some, this represents a sort of entitlement or justification of a life of hard work: "I've worked hard all my life, and now I am hurt, and they owe me." While these may be completely valid and entirely true, unfortunately many of these patients don't realize that within this context, change and healing are not possible. They may be stuck in a pattern of disability and end up suffering forever.

This brings up the problems related to Medicaid patients. With even less income, often on survival level, how can those patients afford the kinds of tests and treatment which we describe in these pages? For the most part, they can't. This raises all sorts of ethical issues that we wrestle with constantly. How can we help those unfortunate patients with little or no money, or can we? I don't have the answers to these questions, but they are important concerns for all of us.

The bottom line here is that each patient needs to search her own heart for her true commitment to healing. The more sincere that desire, the more likely that she will reach her goal. No matter how ill a patient is, I believe that healing is possible. I, of course, do not do the healing. That's between God and my patient. But I can help to provide the hope and the blueprint by which healing may be achieved.

Chapter 26

To Make Things Worse ... or Better

On Suffering as an Attitude Problem

*Y*ou may not be quite ready for this chapter, or perhaps it is exactly the right time for you to read this. However, be aware that it will take courage to fully take in this information and to apply it with complete honesty to yourself. Plus, I think this is really important. So please, take a deep breath and dive in.

Even if you have a severe illness and have been told by experts that "there is nothing else that can be done," it is usually possible to find a wide variety of ways to improve our ability to cope with it. No matter what the medical condition may be, we tend to make it worse (often much worse) by how we view it. Our *attitude* toward the problem profoundly affects our experience of the problem. Whenever we sense that something is wrong, fear enters the picture. Could my illness be really serious? Could I die? Will I suffer? How much will I suffer? How long will it last? Will I be able to keep on working at my job? What will happen to my family? Will I be able to pay the bills? These are unavoidable questions that flood our minds with doubt and fear as soon as we begin to feel poorly. Even a simple cold can begin the process of bringing fear to the table. Understandably, this fear is magnified intensely when the illness we are beginning to come to grips with is cancer, unremitting pain or fatigue, or an autoimmune disease with a long medical name, or the onset of senility or uncontrollable tremors, or autistic symptoms in our beloved little child, or whatever you have that brings these real concerns to mind.

Fear is compounded by our history with those symptoms. If a close relative died of cancer and it was a difficult death accompanied by some of the awful side effects of radiation or chemotherapy, any symptoms that remind us of this history are all the more terrifying. It is not unusual for me to see patients who have a very treatable tumor refuse all conventional medical treatment. They are often under the mistaken impression that their tumor is frighteningly similar to that of their loved one who died so miserably. Fear closes our minds to options for treatment and takes on a life of its own, adding significant weight to our medical burden.

This is the added element of *suffering*. We suffer from our medical condition, and then we *add* to it all of our fear, frustration, anger, irritability, feelings of loss, abandonment (by family and by God), hopelessness, and despair. These added feelings are not necessarily based on what is actually happening in this very moment, but on our worries about what *might* happen or *could* happen some time in the future. Dwelling on the past and on what we used to be able to do before we got sick, or when we used to be healthy, or active, or loved, or when life was good, serves very little purpose. Living in the past only pushes us to make comparisons that have no value. Yes, when we were twenty, we were stronger, more physically fit, had more stamina, and perhaps had more hair. That may have been ten, twenty, thirty, or forty years ago. But life has moved along, and hopefully we have moved along with it. To bemoan the past only brings a huge dimension of suffering to our current problems. If we can let go of those comparisons, and live in the present, we can eliminate that dimension of suffering we carry with us and truly decrease our current pain and worry. Similarly, if we dwell on our fears about what might happen next, this also adds enormously to our burden of suffering.

A wonderful example of what can happen when you deal with this fear comes from my friend and teacher, Jim Jealous, D.O. Twenty years ago, Jim was diagnosed with cancer of the thyroid gland. "There was a hard nodule on the right side (of his thyroid) and every time I touched it I was very frightened." He felt certain that he could not be healed until he had mastered his fears about what might happen next. So instead of choosing surgery immediately, which is what most people would do, Jim wrestled with his fears for the next year and a half, until he felt that he was no longer controlled by them. At that point, to his surprise, when the thyroid was re-biopsied, the cancer was completely gone and never returned.

Another example is that of Ginny Morgan, a superb teacher of insight meditation. She developed breast cancer and went through the usual treatments of surgery, followed by radiation and chemotherapy. Her first rounds of treatment were very difficult and accompanied by intense nausea, throwing up, loss of appetite, hair loss, and lots of pain and fatigue. As she applied her knowledge of meditation to her treatment, she recognized how she was adding to the difficulty of her experience by not being aware of how her fear and anger and frustration had become a part of her world. As she learned to let go of those future-based thoughts and ideas ("What will happen to me if. . ."), many of her symptoms decreased, and in fact disappeared. The cancer had not been cured, but her suffering from it had diminished greatly. When it recurred several years later, and was found to have metastasized to her spine, her oncologist was astonished to discover that she was not in any pain. This was not a magical cure, but was the result of her awareness of how she added to her suffering when she brought the past and the future into the present moment. Years later, although she still has her cancer, she remains upbeat and maintains a very active teaching schedule. She spends happy hours with her family and is a living inspiration and demonstration of how the correct attitude toward illness can enrich one's life immeasurably.

This is a phenomenon that I see every day. To some extent, every person who becomes ill has to struggle with the way in which they may add to their suffering by their own reaction to illness. Sometimes these attitudes are familial or cultural. When I worked in Minnesota, which has a large Scandinavian population, it was clear that "being strong," a form of stoicism, is a deeply ingrained part of that culture. While it is not true, of course, that everyone of Scandinavian descent feels this way, there was still an intense cultural value that was taught at an early age to not give in to emotional expression as a sign of weakness. Under many circumstances, this attitude can be useful. However, if a suffering human being needs to express her emotion in order to release it, and cannot do so because of cultural restraint, this can add to her burden.

Many people are not aware that emotional energy is contained and held directly in our musculoskeletal system. Yes, the memories of our emotions are held in our minds, but the actual experience of emotion, if not released, moves into the weakest areas of our muscles and fascia (the connective tissue wrapping of our muscles). What I am saying here is that unreleased emotion remains in our bodies, not in our minds, and adds directly to the burden of pain and suffering we are experiencing. Unless we understand this principle and allow some form of release to occur, it will not simply go away. Time alone cannot cure it.

In clinical practice we often see the presence of this emotional backlog when there is a sudden release of tension from the muscle, when that muscle is being treated. While this is a *physical* release when the muscle finally lets go, sometimes an unexpected flow of intense emotion occurs, often accompanied by a memory of when that emotion was first acquired. Massage therapists and acupuncturists see this with some regularity. I have referred to this information in Chapter 17, but it is so important that I think it bears repeating. It helps to understand this phenomena, as otherwise the patient will become afraid, or upset by her experience, and further attempt to repress it by tightening up the muscles she needs to release. Commonly we see the presence of shaking or tremors accompany this release, which simply represents the body's need to release the stored tension. If this emotional release, with or without shaking and tremor, is allowed to occur, this can be a healing experience—but if suppressed, it can make patients feel even worse. We all have our own bodily areas where we are predisposed to store this tension, such as the neck and shoulders, stomach, bronchial tubes, and lower back. This can then be directly related to the onset of headaches, ulcers, asthma, and back pain, and of course much more.

The key to using this information is to be really honest with yourself about your feelings about your illness. Are you making it worse by allowing yourself to dwell on your worries? Following a long discussion of this subject, one of my patients recently returned to our office, thrilled to realize that her self pity had played a major part in her symptoms. When she fully acknowledged and owned her self pity and turned her worries over to God, her irritable bowel disease and bronchospasm improved almost overnight. A wonderful book on this material is Byron Katie's *Loving What Is*, which contains a very clear outline and method of how to analyze these forces in your life.

You can do this. You can search your mind, by praying or meditating, or just being quiet, and discover how you are adding to your suffering . . . and let it go. It is extremely important that you do this, because sometimes we can't heal otherwise.

Recently, a young woman came into my practice with another presentation worthy of our discussion. Although she had not yet graduated from college, she had already seen a vast array of healers of all kinds. She had significant constant pain across her neck and shoulders and down her back. She had had extensive physical therapy, massages of every type and description, extensive prolotherapy, requiring long regular plane trips to another city, and repeated x-rays and MRI scans which failed to provide a treatable cause for her pain. After several visits and treatment with osteopathic manipulation, which produced only fleeting benefit, she expressed the desire to be treated much more frequently as perhaps that might help. We squeezed her into our busy schedule, but somehow it was never convenient for her to make those visits and she cancelled them all at the last minute. At that point, I declined to offer her further visits, as I felt she was the youngest *notcher* I had yet encountered. The word *notcher* is my own term for these patients, who, like the gunslingers of the Old West, put a notch in their belt for every medical encounter they have that doesn't help them. While not common, several times a year patients will appear in my office with a complex story, and they appear to be much more concerned with *telling* that story than with getting any help with their medical condition.

What distinguished this young woman from other notchers were her age and arrogance. As she related her story, she clearly couldn't be bothered to recall the names of any of the physicians or health practitioners she had seen. Like other patients who exhibit this odd behavior, eventually it becomes clear that they are much more interested in proving that you (and nobody else, either) can't help them than in making any progress. This response to treatment is so unusual that it took a long time for me to realize the value of this behavior for these patients. Initially, it made no sense to me. Why would anyone continue to suffer, and sabotage all efforts at treatment, for which they were paying? It took a while, but I finally understood that for these unfortunate individuals, this lack of progress demonstrated, once again, that no one can help them, and they are reaffirming in their own minds how really special and unique they are. Getting better, for them, becomes of secondary importance.

When I worked at the Shealy Institute, where Dr. Norman Shealy was quite well known for his advanced ideas in the treatment of pain and depression, we would occasionally receive these visits. At first, I didn't understand what was happening, but after a while it began to make sense.

Patients would arrive from a distant city, and as they presented their history to us, it was filled with long descriptions of all the famous people they'd seen and how unsuccessful those visits had been. Initially, we would work really hard to help them, only to find that nothing worked. Then, they would trundle off, almost happy, now that they had once again been unable to be helped by yet another famous clinic. By appearing to work with us, and not improving, they were demonstrating to themselves that they were so unique that no one, not even the best clinicians, could help them. After a while, we learned to recognize this behavior early in their presentation, by the long but dearly held litany of all the wonderful doctors who had failed to help them. I learned to respond to this by the end of our interview by sadly shaking my head and commiserating with them: Yes, they were unique and special and way too complicated for us to help them. Paradoxically, they would smile at this and happily wander off, delighted that they could add yet another famous clinic to their list that proved, beyond doubt, how special they and their illness were.

The underlying thought process here runs something like this: "You probably can't help me (after all, no one else has), but I will show up and see what you can do." Alas, showing up is not enough. Unless each patient is personally involved in his healing process, I, Neil Nathan, can't cure him. God can, but only if the individual embraces his role in the illness. At best, I am a catalyst, or helper, to enable the patient to access his own healing resources.

It is always a concern when we think someone may be a notcher that we may be guilty of arrogance ourselves. We must always remain aware that maybe, just maybe, we are missing a rare diagnosis and not doing right by that patient. We must always come to the table with as much humility as we can genuinely muster.

Each patient must, therefore, search her own heart for the deepest truths about her own attitudes toward healing. While sometimes that part of her journey is the most difficult, it may also be the most rewarding. Healing requires not just hope, but also commitment and dedication.

Further Reading

Chodron, Pema. *When Things Fall Apart: Heart Advice for Difficult Times.* Boston: Shambhala, 1997.

Katie, Byron. *Loving What Is.* New York: Three Rivers, 2002.

Kornfield, Jack. *A Path with Heart.* New York: Bantam, 1993.

❖ ❖ ❖

Chapter 27

One More for the Road

The Most Valuable Thing I've Ever Done

When it comes to the emotional and spiritual components of healing, words often cannot adequately communicate what we are feeling.

I'd like to end this book with a story from my early experiences in medical practice. Even now, years later, I look back on this moment as perhaps my finest "work," although in reality, I cannot know how this event was perceived by others. I just know how I felt, and, hopefully, that is sufficient.

In the fall of 1985, while working in private practice in Duluth, Minnesota, I was asked by my colleagues in another clinic to cover for them for just a few hours while they held their annual Labor Day picnic for their clinic staff and families. I readily agreed to provide coverage but was surprised when a local emergency room called me but a few minutes after they'd signed out to me. An elderly gentleman, a longtime patient of one of my colleagues, had just presented to the emergency room in severe cardiac failure, and they were admitting him to the hospital. I immediately ran over to the hospital, where cardiologists had taken over the intensive care procedures and were trying to revive him and save his life. Unfortunately, his heart attack had been a massive one, and after a valiant attempt at resuscitation, this gentleman died.

His wife was sitting anxiously in the waiting area of the intensive care unit, her hands clasped together, a look of great distress upon her face. I was uncertain how to approach her; after all, I didn't know her husband, and during his intense resuscitation, we never even had the chance to exchange a few words. How could I comfort her? She did not know me, and I could not honestly provide even a few platitudes about her husband, whom I had not known. I was lost for words. I had no idea what to do. I only knew that she was dreadfully upset and needed comforting.

So I sat down next to her, explained who I was, how I came to be there, and what had happened to her husband. Not knowing what else to do, I took her hand and held it for a moment. There was nothing more to say. She seemed reluctant for me to pull my hand away, so I just sat with her, holding her hand. Time passed, and when I finally patted her hand and stood up to say goodbye, I was astonished that two hours had passed.

Although I had, to all intents and purposes, done almost nothing during these hours, I left the hospital feeling that I had truly been of service that day. I still feel that this may have been the most valuable thing I've ever done in my thirty-eight years of medical practice.

Sometimes we get caught up in the details of medical practice, and we get wrapped up in all of the technology and the chemistry and the multi-syllabic words and difficult-to-pronounce names. And sometimes, life reminds us that we are, essentially, only human, and that it is our caring for others that is our finest gift.

Postscript

More Hope for Healing

I would like to leave you with some cutting-edge, hot-off-the-presses vignettes that reflect my realistic hope that additional healing is just around the corner. My colleagues from around the globe are hard at work, delving into the problems of chronic illness, and some very exciting new research has just emerged that gives us glimpses into where our next breakthroughs may come from.

Paul Cheney, M.D., Ph.D., from Asheville, North Carolina, has been a pioneer in the field of chronic fatigue since his initial involvement with the Incline Village, Nevada, epidemic which occurred in the late 1980s. With Paul's long-standing interest and expertise in this area, his practice, like ours, has gravitated toward seeing the sickest patients. In fact, Paul's patients tend to be so compromised that he has identified an even deeper level of dysfunction in some of them, a level below the one we characteristically evaluate. Paul has noticed that as chronic fatigue worsens, the body chemistry becomes so dysfunctional that patients' systems cannot tolerate oxygen as others can. Dr. Cheney calls them *oxygen toxic*. Using carefully performed Echocardiography studies he has demonstrated this difficulty with many of his patients. As his investigations have continued, he has come to believe that the delicate enzyme systems in the liver, called the P-450 electron chain, cannot function properly, and that the fatigue experienced by these unfortunate individuals actually represents an *adaptive* response on their part to try to prevent their bodies from getting an excessive amount of oxygen, which could further harm them.

The good news is that Paul has recently discovered what he calls "cell-signaling factors," which, when applied transdermally (to the skin) on a regular basis, allows these patients to improve dramatically. We have just begun utilizing these materials with several of our patients and we eagerly await the opportunity to evaluate the results of this new treatment.

Ritchie Shoemaker, M.D., from Pokemoke, Maryland, has recently had the opportunity to test the newly available nasal spray Vasoactive Intestinal Peptide (VIP) on his severely compromised mold patients. VIP is an important chemical produced by specific brain areas, and mold-toxic patients lose the ability to manufacture it in adequate amounts. In a pilot study of sixty such patients, fifty-nine have demonstrated significant clinical improvement. We are scheduled to embark on a more elaborate pilot study with Dr. Shoemaker to further study the potential benefits of VIP in our sickest patients.

Speaking of VIP, Mario Delgado, Ph.D., from Granda, Spain, and Doina Ganea, Ph.D., at Temple University in Philadelphia, a long-term colleague of Dr. Delgado's, have recently completed a study of the benefits of VIP for patients with sarcoidosis. They are already involved in clinical trials for evaluating its use in other autoimmune diseases, as well.

While the re-discovery of the importance of vitamin D is ongoing, and many physicians are now testing vitamin D levels and treating them aggressively. Dr. Eugene Shippen, M.D., from Wyomissing, Pennsylvania, has recently reviewed the available research data that suggests that vitamin D is a key player in healing a compromised immune system. For many years, we have prescribed only 400 IU daily of that vitamin for most of our patients, without taking into consideration our concurrent recommendations for sunscreen use for preventing skin cancers. As most of the vitamin D we need is made by our skin in response to its interaction with sunlight, and sunscreens block 97 percent of vitamin D formation in our bodies, we are now seeing a virtual epidemic of vitamin D deficiency.

While we have long recognized the importance of vitamin D's role in allowing us to adequately absorb calcium into our bodies and build strong bones, we were unaware, until recently, of how important that vitamin is in regulating the function of our immune system. We have also realized that the dosage of vitamin D previously recommended was quite inadequate, and we are now using 4000-5000 IU daily, with even more for those with measured low levels of that vitamin. Dr. Shippen has emphasized that improving 25-hydroxy-vitamin D (the preferred form of measurement) blood levels to between 50 and 80 ng/mL is optimal, especially for those with autoimmune diseases. He has recently published a ground-breaking protocol for the treatment of endometriosis which has added a whole new dimension to our approach.

Jacob Teitelbaum, M.D., now living in Hawaii, has recently completed a study of the use of D-ribose in the treatment of chronic fatigue and fibromyalgia, demonstrating benefits in up to 70 percent of his patients. Using a dose of 5 gm (one scoop) of D-ribose dissolved in water three times a day appears optimal. At Jacob's urging, I have used this in my practice for the past year and confirm the benefits he has described.

Allesio Fasano, M.D., at the University of Maryland School of Medicine, has just completed his research into the chemistry of the "tight junctions" between intestinal cells, which we have discussed as so important in limiting bowel damage and the onset of food allergy. He has identified a natural molecule called *zonulin*, which controls the permeability through those tight junctions. Additionally, Dr. Fasano has worked with the development of a medication called *Larotozide acetate*, which is currently being used in clinical trials. These trials give us great hope that new treatments will soon be available.

Liv Bode, Ph.D., and Hanns Ludwig, D.V.M., Ph.D., Professors at the Free University of Berlin, have been able to identify a unique RNA virus that appears to be present in a high percentage of patients with chronic fatigue and depression. The virus, called *Bornavirus*, is transmitted to humans primarily through contact with horses, although animals, such as cats, can transmit it as well. In horses, this virus induces apathy, somnolence, movement disorders, and loss of appetite. In humans, it is associated with chronic fatigue, depression, obsessive compulsive disorders, hyperactivity, and Alzheimer's disease. They have developed blood tests to allow us to make the diagnoses, and those tests should be available for our use, shortly. Even more exciting, they have done several studies showing that an anti-viral medication, Amantidine, given in doses of 100-200 mg, twice daily, can be curative if given for long periods of time.

I have utilized this treatment in several of my more severely depressed patients who had not responded to conventional medications and who had known exposure to horses. I noted significant improvement in four of the first five patients I treated. Liv and Hanns's work underscores our increasing awareness that many so-called psychological conditions may actually be caused by micro-organisms, and it also provides realistic hope for new treatments as our knowledge evolves.

Still on the subject of infectious agents, Kenny DeMeirleir, M.D., Ph.D., at the University of Brussels in Belgium, has recently completed a study that underscores an awareness that several species of the *Strep* bacteria, commonly found in the intestinal tract and long-assumed to be benign, may not be. He has provided the antibiotic Cipro, in doses of 500 mg twice daily for one week, monthly for three months, for patients who have these bacteria noted on stool testing. He reports marked improvement in thirty-eight of fifty-eight patients with chronic fatigue and fibromyalgia. I anticipate working with Dr. DeMeirleir to expand this study in the near future.

Additional exciting research on the role of infectious agents as possible contributors to the cause of chronic fatigue comes from Lawrence Klapow, Ph.D., from Santa Rosa, California, who has spent the last fifteen years identifying and clarifying our knowledge of an unusual roundworm parasite called *Cryptostrongyloides pulmoni*. Patients infected with this roundworm typically have a low grade eosinophilia (a cell normally evaluated on a common CBC, or complete blood count) and a rash, in addition to their fatigue. Dr. Klapow has recently discovered that fourteen of thirty patients with chronic fatigue were infested with this parasite, which can be diagnosed by the careful evaluation of naturally expressed sputum from the lung (where the parasite resides). Early studies indicate that treatment of this parasite with several medications, including inhaled Ivermectin and Thiobendazole, may be effective over many months, giving us great hope that new diagnostic approaches and treatments will be helpful.

Hot off the presses is the research of Judy Mikovits and her colleagues, who published an article in the October 8, 2009 issue of *Science* titled, "Detection of an Infectious Retrovirus, XMRV, in Blood Cells of Patients with Chronic Fatigue Syndrome." Utilizing elegant scientific techniques, this paper is the first to strongly demonstrate the presence of a newly identified virus as a significant contributor to Chronic Fatigue Syndrome. This finding will greatly expand our ability to understand, and to diagnose and treat this condition.

In the field of pain management, whole books have been devoted to the uses of a variety of electrical devices for treatment. The TENS machine has been in use since its development by Dr. Norman Shealy in the late 1970s. It typically operates at frequencies between 2 and 200 Hz. Saul Liss, Ph.D., subsequently developed the CES (Cranial Electrical Stimulator) for use at frequencies at 15,000 Hz, which expanded the uses of TENS into applications on the head region, leading to progress in the treatment of depression, fatigue, and headaches.

Newer and exciting developments in the field of electrical stimulation involve the use of frequency-specific microcurrent devices, which operate in the range of 10-500 microamperes (a millionth of an ampere). Using carefully prescribed frequencies can address the healing of scar tissue and the immune system as well as a wide variety of pain syndromes. This technique utilizes the newly delineated concept that cells communicate with each other electrically, and that by finding and stimulating these frequencies, we may literally be able to "reset" the nervous system and thereby treat a variety of conditions that were previously resistant to a variety of medical approaches.

Along similar lines, the Scenar device, developed in Russia and promoted by Australian researchers, uses tiny amounts of electricity over painful areas of the body, and measures how the body receives that energy in a feedback mechanism that allows the machine to alter the pattern of energy that is delivered—which again allows us to "reset" the nervous system.

Lee Cowden, M.D., from Chandler, Arizona, and currently President of the Academy of Bio-Energetic and Integrative Medicine, has recently combined some of this technology. Utilizing the newer-generation electrodermal screening tests, he creates a unique energetic "fingerprint" which can be placed in the form of a solution for each patient, and then passes a LED light through that solution onto the patient, to assist that individual in both detoxification and healing. We have observed some astonishing successes using this technique with some of our most challenging patients.

These vignettes are only a tiny part of the research that is ongoing, and I present them to you to whet your appetite for learning more as these fields of knowledge unfold. All of them, I trust, reflect my main message: There is HOPE.

Further Reading

Fasano, Alessio. "Biological Perspectives: Physiological, Pathological, and Therapeutic Implications of Zonulin-Mediated Intestinal Barrier Modulation." *The American Journal of Pathology* 173.5 (2008): 1-9.

Gonzalez-Rey, Elena, and Mario Delgado. "Vasoactive intestinal peptide and regulatory T-cell induction: a new mechanism and therapeutic potential for immune homeostasis." *Trends in Molecular Medicine* 13.6 (2007): 241-251.

❖ ❖ ❖

Appendix

Medical Conditions Discussed in the Case Histories

Case History	Chapter	Condition(s) Discussed
Travis's Story	Chapter 3	Adrenal (DHEA) deficiency, persistent rib cage pain
Karen's Story	Chapter 3	Fibromyalgia/chronic fatigue, adrenal (DHEA) deficiency
Carla's Story	Chapter 3	Fibromyalgia/chronic fatigue, adrenal deficiency (DHEA, cortisol, mineralocorticoids)
Jim's Story	Chapter 4	Magnesium deficiency
Tanya's Story	Chapter 5	Wilson's syndrome, fibromyalgia/chronic fatigue
Ellie's Story	Chapter 5	Wilson's syndrome, chronic fatigue
Estelle's Story	Chapter 5	Iodine deficiency, fibromyalgia/chronic fatigue
Kristy's Story	Chapter 6	Estrogen deficiency, fibromyalgia/chronic fatigue, adrenal deficiency (DHEA)
Sheldon's Story	Chapter 6	Testosterone deficiency, chronic fatigue
Clarence's Story	Chapter 7	Food allergy and joint pain
Olivia's Story	Chapter 7	Food allergy and inflammatory bowel disease (Crohn's)
Norma's Story	Chapter 7	Food allergy and rheumatoid arthritis
Rochelle's Story	Chapter 8	Dysbiosis and irritable bowel syndrome (IBS)

CASE HISTORY	CHAPTER	CONDITION(S) DISCUSSED
Nathan's Story	Chapter 8	Food allergy and failure to thrive, bronchospasm (asthma), eczema
Karl's Story	Chapter 9	Hypoglycemia, chronic fatigue and depression
Ed's Story	Chapter 10	Mercury toxicity, chronic fatigue, cognitive dysfunction
Patrick's Story	Chapter 10	Root canal, hypertension, cognitive dysfunction, weakness, shoulder pain
Maureen's Story	Chapter 11	Mold toxicity, severe nausea, mood swings, cognitive dysfunction, Multiple Chemical Sensitivities (MCS), headaches
Barbara's Story	Chapter 11	Mold toxicity, seizures, migraines, cognitive dysfunction, numbness and tingling (paresthesias)
Mark's Story	Chapter 12	Chronic Lyme disease, headaches, fatigue, cognitive dysfunction
Kendra's Story	Chapter 12	Chronic EBV (Epstein-Barr Syndrome), chronic fatigue, cognitive dysfunction
Hallie's Story	Chapter 12	Chronic EBV, fibromyalgia
Katy's Story	Chapter 13	Amino acid deficiencies, fibromyalgia
Bernice's Story	Chapter 13	Amino acid deficiencies, Parkinson's disease
Edward's Story	Chapter 14	Methylation chemistry dysfunction, chronic fatigue, Wilson's syndrome, cortisol deficiency, DHEA deficiency, magnesium deficiency

CASE HISTORY	CHAPTER	CONDITION(S) DISCUSSED
Henry's Story	Chapter 15	Sciatica from Pyriformis syndrome, trigger point therapy
Heidi's Story	Chapter 17	Chronic facial pain, craniosacral manipulation
Kristina's Story	Chapter 18	Chronic low back (sacroiliac) pain, migraine headaches, osteopathic and craniosacral manipulation, prolotherapy
My Story	Chapter 18	Prolotherapy, chronic shoulder pain
Betty's Story	Chapter 18	Prolotherapy, chronic knee pain
Duncan's Story	Chapter 19	Chelation for coronary artery disease
Melvin's Story	Chapter 19	Chelation for coronary artery disease
Natalie's Story	Chapter 19	Chelation for mercury toxicity, cognitive dysfunction
Ingrid's Story	Chapter 21	Ovarian cancer, Livingston vaccines
Isaac's Story	Chapter 22	Autism Spectrum, Defeat Autism Now! approaches
Nina's Story	Chapter 22	ADHD/Absence seizures (Petit Mal)
Calvin's story	Chapter 24	Mold toxicity, cognitive dysfunction, muscles spasms

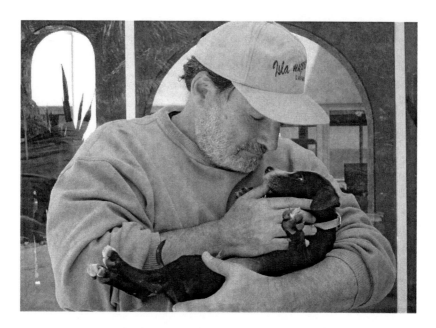

A graduate of The University of Chicago's Pritzker School of Medicine, Dr. Neil Nathan has been practicing medicine for thirty-eight years. He is a Board Certified Family Physician, and has combined his knowledge of conventional medicine with his extensive background in holistic medicine and pain management in his efforts to provide diagnostic and therapeutic hope and healing for those who have, unfortunately, "fallen through the medical cracks."

Dr. Nathan currently resides in northern California with his wife, Cheryl, three dogs, and a cat. He is thoroughly enjoying the opportunity to savor their walks on the beach and through the redwood forests, on an almost daily basis.

He continues to practice medicine, do research, and has more books currently on the word processor. He, and his colleagues who provide the type of medical diagnosis and care described on these pages, can be reached for consultation or appointment at

Gordon Medical Associates
3471 Regional Parkway
Santa Rosa, California, 95403
Phone: 707-575-5180
FAX: 707-575-5509
Email: neil@gordonmedical.com

Index

Eichler

CPSIA information can be obtained at www.ICGtesting.com
Printed in the USA
LVOW061630180312

273591LV00001B/147/P